THE WATER FASTING GUIDE

How to Restore Your Body, Heal Yourself, Feel Better and Lose Weight with Water Fasting

By Emily Moore

Copyright© 2019 by Emily Moore - All rights reserved.

Copyright: No part of this publication may be reproduced without written permission from the author, except by a reviewer who may quote brief passages or reproduce illustrations in a review with appropriate credits; nor may any part of this book be reproduced, stored in a retrieval system, or transmitted in any form or by any means – electronic, mechanical, photocopying, recording, or other – without prior written permission of the copyright holder.

The trademarks are used without any consent, and the publication of the trademark is without permission or backing by the trademark owner. All trademarks and brands within this book are for clarifying purposes only and are owned by the owners themselves.

Disclaimer: The information in this book is not to be used as professional medical advice and is not meant to treat or diagnose medical problems. The information presented should be used in combination with guidance from a competent professional person.

The information in this book is true and complete to the best of our knowledge. All recommendations are made without guarantee on the part of the author. It is the sole responsibility of the reader to educate and train in the use of all or any specialized equipment that may be used or referenced in this book that could cause harm or injury to the user or applicant. The author disclaims any liability in connection with the use of this information. References are provided for informational purposes only and do not constitute endorsement of any websites or other sources. Readers should be aware that the websites listed in this book may change.

First Printing, 2019 - Printed in the United States of America

TABLE OF CONTENTS

Introduction	1
Water Fasting	3
What Do We Know About It?	3
The History of Fasting	5
12 Surprising Water Fasting Facts	6
10 Most Common Fasting Myths Debunked	8
How Does Fasting Work?	11
The Science Behind Water Fasting	13
Why Water Fast?	19
Pros and Cons	22
6 Proven Water Fasting Techniques	23
How to Water Fast – All You Need to Know	25
Research-Backed Guide to Lose 40 Pounds in 30 Days	28
Case Studies	35
5 Safety Tips You Wish You Knew	41
Most Common Mistakes and How to Avoid Them	45
8 Insider Tips to Starting a Fast	49
7 Top Tips for Managing Your Fast	63
Exercise and Water Fasting	72
5 Ultimate Steps for Breaking Your Fast the Right Way	73
10 Guaranteed Tricks for Getting Through Your Water Fast	79

FAQ	81
Conclusion	87
About the Author	89

INTRODUCTION

Water fasting is a type of fasting in which someone only consumes water for a certain period of time. There are a number of reasons that people might do this. Maybe it's to lose weight, maybe it's for the potential health benefits that fasting offers, or maybe it's for religious or spiritual reasons. Whatever your personal reason is, reading this book will give you all of the information that you need to be fully equipped to perform a *successful* fast.

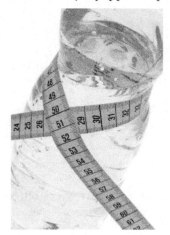

Here are the most common **health benefits** of water fasting:

- *Detoxification* – water fasting helps rid our bodies of waste. An effective fast will make your skin, liver, colon, lymph glands, kidneys, and lungs clear of toxins.

- *Immune System Strength* – during a fast, your body's energy gets redirected from your digestive system to the centers that deal with your metabolism and your immune system, restoring their natural function.

- *Extended Life Expectancy* – all the damaged tissues and major illnesses within the body are repaired, leaving the body rejuvenated and in the optimal state for growth.

- *Healthier Cardiovascular System* – your blood pressure will be stabilized, and your cholesterol levels will be lowered, giving you a much healthier internal system.

- *Improved Skeletal and Muscular Systems* – fasting can stimulate important anti-inflammatory activity in the skeletal and muscular systems, healing from almost all pains, aches, and arthritis in muscles and joints.

- *Weight Loss* – eliminating excess fat will result in weight loss. Water fasting is a great cure for obesity.

- *Increased Self-Control* – if you can stick out to a fast, then you can do anything!

- *Increased Energy* – normally, most of your energy is used on your digestive system. This isn't necessary when you're fasting, giving you more energy to use for other things.

- *Increased Body Sensitivity* – you'll be given a much deeper sense of awareness of your body. The better you know your body, the better you'll be able to treat it in the future.

- *Better Mental Balance* – fasting successfully leaves you feeling much more in control of your emotions and feelings. You'll find a noticeable benefit with this.

If all of this doesn't convince you that water fasting can help you solve your problems, then continue reading to discover just how this method can help you **repair your DNA, increase your energy levels, and lose 40 pounds in 30 days** – who wouldn't want all of these things? And this is one of the best, proven ways to help you achieve this.

This guide is the most extensive on the market, showing you all of the scientific studies that prove just how beneficial fasting can be, the best way to perform a successful fast, and tips and tricks to help you remain motivated throughout. By the time you have finished reading, you'll have everything at your disposal to ensure that your water fast is safe, successful and gives you the results that you desire – whatever your end goal might be.

So, read on and good luck with *your* fasting experience!

WATER FASTING

WHAT DO WE KNOW ABOUT IT?

Fasting is the act of going without food or drink for a set period of time and has been proven to be a beneficial healing method. It is an ancient method, used for spiritual purposes and treating common diseases. An effective period of fasting is essential for every human body.

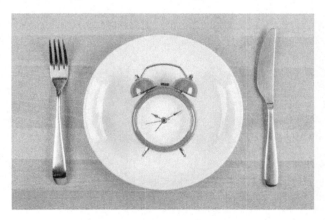

A very popular way of doing this is **water fasting** – which means consuming *only* water for that set amount of time. Water is chosen because it's essential for keeping the human body alive and dehydrated, it contains zero calories, and it has been scientifically hailed for its detoxing qualities.

During your fasting period, the water will absorb all of the toxins that your body needs to excrete, effectively rebooting your system and helping you to absorb nutrients more effectively.

The length of your water fast will depend on your individual and your body's needs. Of course, it's always recommended that you consult a doctor before starting your fast to get the right, most suitable advice for you. Water fasts typically last between 24 hours and 10 days – with 3 days being the *most* common duration.

It has been proven that water fasting is much **more successful than juice fasting**. It gives your digestive system a much-needed rest, while also cleaning out your system. It also gives you a physical and emotional rest because of its therapeutic effects on your body. This will be demonstrated much more clearly as we go through the following chapters.

The History Of Fasting

You can't actually pinpoint a beginning of fasting because it's been happening forever — even in the animal world before humans started walking the planet. Animals abstain from food when they're stressed, unwell, and even sometimes when they feel the slightest unease. It's a natural reaction for them, a tendency that helps them find balance, rest, and the ability to conserve energy during distressing times.

Herbert Shelton was a physician who supervised more than 40,000 fasts. From that experience, he wrote, *"Fasting must be recognized as a fundamental and radical process that is older than any other mode of caring for the sick organism, for it is employed on the plane of instinct..."*

There is a reason that the great early philosophers and healers, such as Galen, Hippocrates, Socrates, Plato, and Aristotle, praised fasting and used it for a health and healing therapy. Paracelsus is considered one of the fathers of Western medicine, and he is quoted as saying, *"Fasting is the greatest remedy — the physician within."* This means that you can actually use fasting as a way of healing yourself.

It isn't just philosophers that have used fasting for rejuvenation. It's a very common spiritual practice that's used by many varying religions during rites and ceremonies. These are still taking place within the major religions of Judaism, Gnosticism, Hinduism, Islam, Christianity, Buddhism, and the North and South American Indian traditions; commonly occurring during the fall and spring equinoxes. Although this may be for different reasons — purification, spiritual vision, penance, mourning, or sacrifice, to name just a few — some faiths will encourage regular fasting to break or prevent the habit of overeating.

Yoga practices also often include fasting, which dates back over centuries. Paramahansa Yogananda, an Indian yogi and guru, is known to have said, *"Fasting is a natural method of healing."* This methodology is undertaken by alternative health practitioners today — although it's increasingly becoming accepted as a healing method by traditional medicine.

12 Surprising Water Fasting Facts

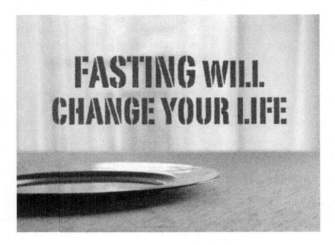

We have looked a little into the benefits of water fasting, but **here are some facts about what it can do for you** that you may not have already known about:

- People always expect to be extremely hungry during their water fast, then are surprised to discover just how quickly the physical sensations of hunger disappear. It's the cravings that stick around for longer. Avoiding temptation will help you stick to your fast.

- Fasting breaks down the body's fat reserves, ridding your body of toxins. This detox will help you feel much happier, healthier, and more energetic.

- Water fasting will leave your digestive and elimination system invigorated, giving your metabolism a chance to speed up.

- Fasting alleviates inflammatory and allergic reactions, such as rheumatoid arthritis, hay fever, and asthma, respectively.

- Fasting can help the body break down, and then recycle, parts of cells that are "old" and could become dangerous. This is called autophagy.

- Fasting assists the body in relieving atypical fluid accumulations that can occur in the legs, ankles, and abdomen.

- Fasting will normalize blood pressure — with the effects lasting much longer than the fast itself, if the faster continues to eat much healthier and exercise accordingly. This means high blood pressure sufferers can then do without their medication.

- Fasting can help the faster overcome addictions and bad habits, such as tobacco, alcohol, and substance abuse. This is because the detox rids the body of the substance that the body is addicted to.

- Fasting can help to clear acne and leave the whites of your eyes looking clearer and brighter — looking better can help you feel better!

- Fasting can restore your taste buds and the taste for healthy food, and detoxifying this way can modify what you crave, reducing the desire for processed or sugary foods.

- Fasting can enhance the function of your other senses, such as vision, hearing, or smell.

- Fasting can give you the perfect gateway and sustain your motivation to making a fresh start. Sometimes, this kick-start is all you need to make a positive lifestyle change.

10 Most Common Fasting Myths Debunked

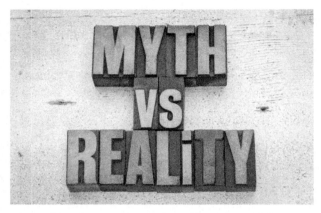

There are a lot of myths out there about fasting, which can easily be debunked by scientific proof. Here are some of the most popular myths:

Myth 1: Fasting is starving

People will typically call "not eating" starving; there is a stark difference between the two. When you fast, your body is consuming its reserves, whereas if you're starving, all your body's reserves have been consumed and the body is living only on its vital tissue, taking muscle first.

This is the reason that our bodies have fat cells to store fuel for when food is scarce – the human body is well-equipped for emergencies where getting sustenance right away isn't possible. The average person actually has enough reserves to last 6 to 8 weeks, if resting. Obviously, this ends up being less because we have to move about – but knowing this information often helps people get through difficult times.

Body fat is necessary, but only about 3% is essential for survival. Most people today have nearly 7 to 10 times this amount – which is excess and a storing place for toxins. Only by breaking this fat down, can we eliminate these toxins from our bodies.

Myth 2: Nutrients are essential for the healing process

As we break down fat, the nutrients make their way into our bloodstreams, where they are available for our bodies to reuse. This means we still get virtually *everything* that we need during fasting. Deficiencies and imbalances are extremely unlikely. In fact, you're more likely to have your nutrient levels corrected rather than thrown out of whack.

Myth 3: Our bodies aren't really *that* toxic

Unfortunately, this isn't true. Our lifestyle choices burden our bodies increasingly over time and make it difficult for our systems to eliminate waste on a regular basis. This often means body cells are getting surrounded by waste, and this has a negative impact on their ability to function correctly. Fasting is essential to overcome this.

Myth 4: Fasting is *only* for the healthy

This just isn't the case at all. It may seem illogical for those who are weak or sick to fast, but the healing benefits work most effectively for them. As long as you consult the advice of a doctor to confirm that you are able to fast, there is nothing that can hold you back. Self-healing in this way is one of the most powerful tools at your disposal.

Myth 5: Fasting makes well people sick

People often mistake the symptoms of fasting as sickness. This isn't a result of the fast, but more of the toxins leaving your body. Any cleanse has the risk of making you feel under the weather at the time – but after all of the nastiness has left your system, you will feel so much better. These symptoms can be headaches, feverishness, sickness – but all of that is ok. Accepting that this may happen will make it much less alarming if it does.

Myth 6: Fasting makes the body detoxify too rapidly

It's often forgotten just how intelligent our bodies are with regards to its own processes. Your body will manage the detoxification process as it sees fit – even at an increased pace. Although you may feel discomfort and side effects, this doesn't mean your body is working overtime.

Myth 7: Colon therapy is essential to avoid auto-intoxication

This myth is based around the theory that everything is dumped near the colon, and that whatever is dumped will end up back in the bloodstream when it isn't excreted. However, it seems that most people carry anywhere between 5 and 10 pounds of waste in their digestive tract, often sitting for months, or even years. To get personalized advice on whether you need to flush this out or not, it's best to consult your doctor. Some people need to do this; some people prefer to do this. It just isn't essential for everyone.

Myth 8: Many conditions contradict fasting

There are actually very few people who cannot fast. Even people with most underlying health conditions can fast with a lot of rest and the supervision of a professional. Consult a health professional for advice to confirm that you aren't one of the very few who cannot fast.

Myth 9: Juice fasting can be a more effective method to fast

Juices are food with caloric content, which means using them to fast is gentler, but a less effective method. When we juice fast, our bodies direct an excessive amount of energy to push those calories through the system, which means a lot less energy is available for healing and cleansing.

Myth 10: Restore your health with fasting alone

Ok, this is less of a myth and more of a message. Fasting does a great deal of the work – but it's only the first step. You also need to eat well and exercise after you have finished the fast – this is the *only* way to maintain the benefits.

Fasting is the first rung on the ladder to a more positive lifestyle change – but it does make the rest of it much easier. Remember, if you can survive on water alone for an extended period of time – you really can do anything!

THE WATER FASTING GUIDE

How Does Fasting Work?

Our bodies go through a certain process when we fast, as explained below.

The Four Phases of Fasting

	Phases	gastrointestinal glycogenolysis				gluconeogenesis				ketosis			
	Fasting Days	1	2	3	4	5	6	7	8	9	10	11	12	13
Energy Source	Glucose													
	Glycogen													
	Amino Acids (Protein)													
	Fatty Acids (Fat)													
	Ketones												Cridland, 1986	

Normally, our bodies turn food into *glucose* – which becomes our primary source of energy. During a fast, we are deprived of this. After the first 24 hours of the fast, our bodies have depleted all of the glucose that we have stored and we switch to 'ketosis,' a state where the body uses its fatty and amino acids as fuel.

This **ketone process** can last 2-3 more days, then the body will start conserving protein in large amounts. Where vital organs and muscle tissue can be protected during extended food deprivation, which would otherwise cause damage. If you fast for more than one week, the body will begin targeting any other non-body protein sources for fuel, typically, nonessential cellular masses, such as degenerative tissues, bacteria, or viruses.

While you're fasting, similar to sleeping, the body focuses on regenerating damaged tissues and removing toxins. Therefore, it is believed that if fasting leads to ketosis and conservation of protein, this evolutionary development can enhance and protect your system from damage during times when food availability is scarce.

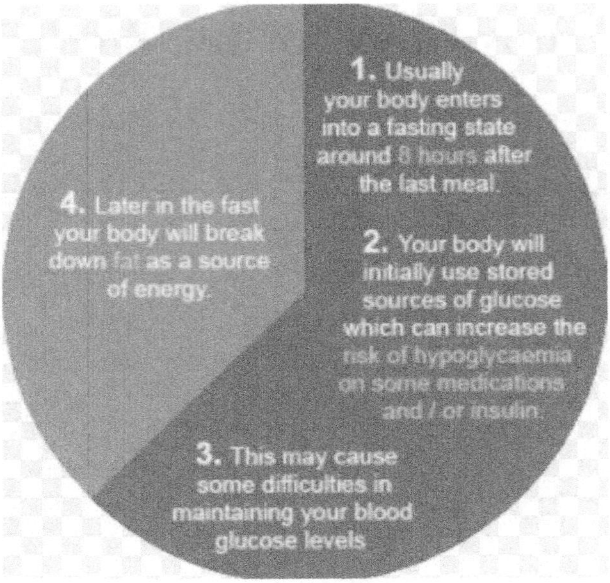
1. Usually your body enters into a fasting state around 8 hours after the last meal.
2. Your body will initially use stored sources of glucose which can increase the risk of hypoglycaemia on some medications and / or insulin.
3. This may cause some difficulties in maintaining your blood glucose levels
4. Later in the fast your body will break down fat as a source of energy.

The Science Behind Water Fasting

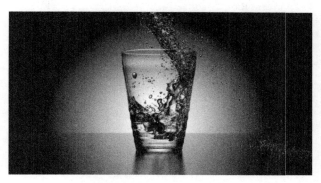

Health Science at *www.healthscience.org* presents the most recent scientific studies conducted by Dr. Alan Goldhamer, founder of the *TrueNorth Health Center*, who has been working on learning more about the benefits of water fasting.

Despite water fasting being a well-known practice, only a minimal amount of scientific research has been documented explaining its safety and efficiency. The National Health Association (NHA) has made it a goal to produce scientific documentation explaining the safety and advantages of fasting. To meet this need, the NHA has raised money to support Dr. Goldhamer and his research.

With this funding, Dr. Goldhamer and the Health Center staff were able to complete a 12-year study, *Medically Supervised Water-only Fasting in the Treatment of Hypertension*, which appeared in the *Journal of Manipulative and Physiological Therapeutics*. This extensive collection of research explained their positive, exceptional results after treating 174 study participants living with **high blood pressure**. According to those results, water fasting helped reduce blood pressure, which in turn could help prevent other heart-related diseases.

Dr. Goldhamer has also written *The Rediscovery of Water-Only Fasting* to study the benefits of water fasting, including **neuroadaptation** – where your body can adapt to low-salt foods, for example, enhancing the elimination of excess sodium and speeding up the process of adopting a healthier diet.

From his work, there is also *Fasting Is the Answer – What Is the Question?* This paper examines the goals that can be achieved by water fasting. This includes tackling **obesity**, **addictions**, and **autoimmune diseases**. These papers all prove what water fasting can do for you.

Of course, Dr. Goldhamer isn't the only person to have conducted scientific research into water fasting. Here we will look at the scientific evidence supporting what it can do for our bodies:

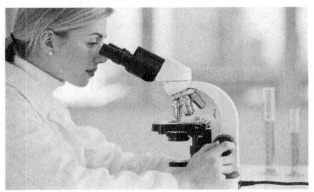

Mental Benefits

Fasting could slow down an age-related decline in motor and cognitive abilities, according to a study from Singh et al., keeping you mentally active for much, much longer. Fasting was proven to delay the onset of a decline in spatial memory and motor skills, as well as hindering the indicators of oxidative stress and mitochondrial dysfunction.

Fasting has also been shown to boost neuronal autophagy in the study conducted by Alirezaei et al. – which helps your brain work at its full capacity. This allows you to function better, think clearer, and keep your brain healthy.

Mood

Many scientists believe that water fasting can clear your mind and really improve your mood. The detox and the internal healing will make you feel much healthier and more energized, which can alleviate the symptoms of depression, as shown by the 2008 Michealson et al. study, which showed a dramatic decrease in depressive and anxiety symptoms in 80% of chronic pain patients.

There is also the Guillaume et al. study, which suggests that a heightened feeling of improved mood, well-being and euphoria, and mental alertness followed a successful bout of fasting – just proving that water fasting can help anyone feel happier.

Brain Health

Fasting has been long thought to help ward off diseases, and a research paper written by Matteson demonstrates that this is certainly true for Alzheimer's and Parkinson's. *"The cells of the brain are put under mild stress that is analogous to the effects of exercise on muscle cells. The overall effect is beneficial."* He believes that fasting gives our brains all that they need to protect themselves from this type of mental decline.

It's also thought that the normalization of your blood sugar levels, that occurs while fasting, will help slow the effects of Huntington's disease. This can be seen in the study conducted by Duan et al.

Immune System

There is no doubt that fasting boosts our immune system. A research paper written by Susan Wu shows that this is because of the regeneration of our white blood cells when we fast. When you go without food, your body wants to conserve energy. One of the ways it does this is by recycling non-essential immune cells, especially damaged cells. What Wu spotted in both the animal and human work is that after prolonged fasting, the white blood cell count decreases. That count bounces back after you break the fast. White blood cells are what help us fight off illness and disease, so the regeneration is extremely useful.

Fat Loss

People often fear that fasting will cause them to feel too hungry to actually lose weight. They worry that they won't be able to stick to it, but the study conducted by Lee et al. shows how fasting actually helps our bodies to produce leptons – making us feel more sated. So, not only will hunger be less of an issue than you first thought, you will also start to learn the signs for when you're *really* hungry, meaning you won't overeat in the future.

If you're interested in learning how much weight you're likely to lose while water fasting, check out *Fasting: The History, Pathophysiology and Complications* which states: *"Early in fasting weight loss is rapid, averaging 0.9 kg per day during the first week and slowing to 0.3 kg per day by the third week; early rapid weight loss is primarily due to negative sodium balance. Metabolically, early fasting is characterized by a high rate of gluconeogenesis with amino acids as the primary substrates. As fasting continues, progressive ketosis develops due to the mobilization and oxidation of fatty acids."*

Longevity

Ensuring that you live a healthy life will help you to live much longer. And fasting can assist you with that aim. For example, the study by Horne et al. proves that fasting can have a positive impact on your heart and should be used as a preventive treatment with the potential to reduce metabolic disease risk.

Another example study comes from Banerjee et al., which looks into how fasting regulates your glucose levels. This allows your digestive system to work in a much more effective manner.

Hormones

Water fasting can have a massive impact on our hormones. An example of this can be seen in the Uchida et al. study, which looks at the impact fasting can have on our growth hormones. It found that after 2 weeks of fasting, there were notable reductions in hepatosomatic index, body weight, and specific growth rate in both females and males.

There is also the thought that fasting can actually help to rebalance our hormones – making us feel much happier and healthier.

Water fasting is also considered a shortcut to DNA repair – which means our body works harder to repair any of the DNA damage that's been done to it. A research paper written by Perkel looks deeper into the way our bodies do this better while being starved. The focus that *would* have been on our digestive system can then be used to do this instead.

Health

Gaian Studies at *www.gaianstudies.org* presents scientific finds that show you exactly what water fasting can do for your health:

- In a hypertension clinical trial, 174 people participated in regulated fasting. The pre-fast lasted 2-3 days, where participants only ate fruits and vegetables. This was followed by a water-only fast lasting 10-11 days. Following that was a 6-7-day post-fast featuring a low-fat, low-sodium vegan diet. Blood pressure was measured in the participants before the trial started and was in excess of 140 millimeters of mercury (mm HG) systolic, 90 diastolic or both. By the trial's end, 90% of participants recorded blood pressure at less than 140/90. In fact, the higher the initial recorded blood pressure was, the farther it dropped. The average drop among participants was 37/13. Participants with stage 3 hypertension (over 180/110) recorded an average reduction of 60/17. Those taking medication prior to fasting were able to stop taking it. A number of similar trials have been recorded, where fasting has proven to be an efficient method for reducing blood pressure and regulating cardiovascular function. Once the fasting is broken, blood pressure tends to remain low.

- Fasting has been considered beneficial in cases of congestive heart failure and chronic cardiovascular disease. It can help reduce atheroma, total cholesterol, and triglycerides and increase HDL levels.

THE WATER FASTING GUIDE

- Fasting has been considered efficient for treating type II diabetes, often permanently reversing the condition.

- Fasting has been considered effective in treating obesity. It has a lasting impact on conditions of obesity, fat stores in the body, metabolism, and leptin.

- Fasting has been considered beneficial in epilepsy, based on certain studies, because it can reduce the severity, length, and number of seizures. It can be especially helpful in easing childhood epilepsy.

- Fasting has been considered an effective medical intervention for acute pancreatitis based on a 1988 clinical trial focused on 88 participants. Cimetidine and nasogastric suction were not found to be as helpful as fasting. Symptoms were relieved by fasting regardless of the disease's etiology.

- Fasting has been considered an effective treatment for both osteo-arthritis and rheumatoid arthritis, because it stimulates anti-inflammatory processes in the body. Researchers determined fasting lowered ESR, alleviated pain and stiffness, arthralgia, and the need for medication.

- Fasting has been considered an effective treatment for autoimmune diseases, such as acute glomerulonephritis, lupus, chronic urticaria, and rosacea.

- Fasting has been considered helpful in treating severely toxic contamination. For example, in some clinical trials, people poisoned by PCB noted experiencing "dramatic" relief after fasting 7-10 days.

- Fasting has been studied as an effective treatment to improve poor immune function. Some studies found that fasting can increase bactericidal and monocyte killing function, macrophage activity, natural killer cell activity, cell-mediated immunity, neutrophil bactericidal activity, and immunoglobulin levels; and decrease antigen-antibody complexes, lymphocyte blastogenesis, and complement factors.

- Fasting has also been considered an efficient treatment for insomnia, psoriasis, multiple sclerosis, eczema, hives, psychosomatic disease, hay fever, depression, allergies, neurosis, gout, schizophrenia, intestinal parasites, neurogenic bladder, uterine fibroids, thrombophlebitis, duodenal ulcers, varicose ulcers, lumbago, fibromyalgia, bronchial asthma, neurocirculatory disease, inflammatory bowel disease, and irritable bowel syndrome.

- Fasting has been found to actually increase our energy levels, allowing our bodies to function more effectively.

- Fasting has long been considered an effective method of increasing a person's life span, and this is beginning to generate support in scientific literature. Partaking in a regular 4-day fast has been found to increase the life span for immunocompromised and normal mice.

- Fasting as a treatment for cancer has sparked debate, however, some data has been produced *showing* how fasting can help prevent cancer. There has been a preventative effect on liver cancer in rats who took part in occasional water fasting (2 days per week).

- While there may not be a lot of research, the papers about water fasting that are written show positive results. As fasting benefits become more obvious, even more studies will be conducted and get published.

Why Water Fast?

So, we have already looked at the many benefits of water fasting – weight loss, health benefits, detoxification, to name just a few – but we can't discuss the reasons people choose to abstain from food without looking at the metabolic boost you'll receive from your water fast. Our metabolism is comprised of the chemicals inside our bodies that determine whether we lose or gain weight, and water fasting causes this to work overtime – clearing out and rebooting our systems.

We need **four main *macronutrients*** to make the metabolism process happen:

- Proteins
- Fats
- Carbohydrates
- Nucleic Acids (found in DNA)

These factors can be found in food, and the **food pyramid** has been created to ensure that we're getting enough of these for our bodies to function as normal.

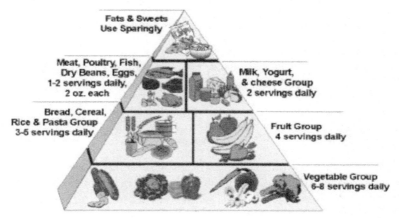

Our **metabolism** then starts to break this food down as follows:

- Proteins become Amino Acids
- Fats become Fatty Acids
- Carbohydrates become Glucose
- Nucleic Acids become Nucleotides

Your body then has three options with what to do with these components:

- Break them down further
- Repair and rebuild them
- Store them for later use

The process begins the moment that we are conceived and doesn't end until we die. It works to allow us to think, to move, to grow – everything is affected by the way that it works. However, there are a lot of **factors that have an impact on how well our metabolism works**, and this includes:

- *Age* – unfortunately, the older you get, the slower your metabolism becomes.
- *Body size* – if you're taller or heavier, your metabolism will need to work much harder to get the job done.
- *Muscle mass* – a higher muscle mass often leads to a more successful metabolism.
- *Gender* – men have a speedier metabolism than women.
- *Activity level* – exercise has a massive impact on the way that your metabolism works. The more you move, the better it will be.
- *Hormonal factors* – certain hormones and related illnesses will affect your metabolism.
- *Genetics* – you should be able to get a glimpse of how your metabolism will work from your family history.
- *Environmental factors* – the weather can actually have an impact on your metabolic rate. If it's very hot or cold, your system needs to work much harder for this process to work.
- *Diet* – eating healthy, only when you're hungry, and at a scheduled time can make your metabolism work more effectively.
- *Drugs* – prescription drugs, caffeine, and nicotine can slow down your metabolism.

This is why water fasting is *so* important. It allows your system to clear itself and reboot. As long as you continue to eat well after your fast, your body will maintain this metabolic boost – assisting you long into the future.

But metabolism isn't the only reason to water fast. One of the other reasons is **weight loss**. It stands to reason that if you aren't consuming any calories, then you *have* to be burning some – no matter how little you're doing.

The typical weight loss for water fasting is approximately *3 pounds per day* – but this will vary from person to person. No matter whether you take part in a long or a short fast, the real important thing to remember is eating right after your fast. That's why **breaking the fast in the right way is so important**, it prevents you from gaining weight after all of your hard work. This is covered later in this book.

Not only is weight loss a side effect of water fasting, so is a speedy **detox**. When you aren't eating anything, your digestive system has a chance to clear itself out of any of the toxins that remain in your bloodstream. This is why you may feel a little unpleasant at times – this isn't the fast, but your body getting rid of all the nastiness inside.

One of the more surprising reasons that people water fast is as a part of **therapy**. While you're clearing out your body of all of its toxins, and allowing it to heal, you will also receive an emotional clarity that you weren't expecting. Water fasting is often referred to as *therapeutic fasting* because it's the most successful method of doing this.

When people fast for **spiritual reasons**, it's to bring them closer to God. You will also feel an energized emotional boost when you water fast – this is true whether you take part in a short- or long-term fast.

Pros And Cons

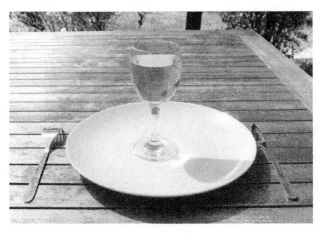

Of course, as with all diets and fasting, there are pros and cons to water fasting. Knowing these and being aware of them can help you make a more informed decision. Here are the most prominent points:

Pros

- It requires no special equipment – just fresh, pure water – so it's very easy to start.
- It can be done at home. Some people prefer to do it under medical supervision, but this isn't essential.
- It cleanses, detoxifies, and purifies the body offering all kinds of amazing health benefits.

Cons

- There are some side effects that you may experience when water fasting. These are listed later in this book.
- A water fast may be difficult for some people to complete.
- There are certain groups of people that should not attempt a water fast – always consult a doctor beforehand to ensure that you are not one of them.

If you have any concerns at all, it is always recommended that you speak to a health professional before undertaking a fast. That way you can get advice that's personalized to you and your situation.

6 Proven
Water Fasting Techniques

There are many different ways that you can perform a water fast. All these types of fasting will offer you benefits; it's up to you to select one that suits your individual needs, your lifestyle requirements, and your end goal.

1. Dry Fasting

This fast is the most extreme and often called the *Absolute Fast*. The roots of dry fasting are spiritual and consists of foregoing water and food for short periods. We do not necessarily recommend this, as it is really only for very experienced fasters.

2. Liquid Fasting

This is fasting using only liquids – no food is consumed whatsoever. This can be any liquid or can be more specific as shown by the types of fast that follow.

3. Juice Fasting

This fast includes some nutritional value just in a pure, or natural, form and is very popular. This is because almost any vegetable, fruit, or juice can be blended with the powerful juicers that are currently on the market.

4. Water Fasting

This fast may be the oldest of its kind and is thought to provide the greatest physically therapeutic benefit in a shorter period of time, because the detox-ification process happens quickly. Water fasting is also the easiest type of liquid fasting.

5. Master Cleanse

This is a relatively new method, which is often called the *Lemonade Diet*. The Master Cleanse uses a recipe that includes pure maple syrup. Intestinal cleansing is a major aspect of this methodology.

Master Cleanse Recipe

Combine:

- 8 oz purified water

- 2 tbl lime or lemon juice, fresh squeezed

- 2 tbl maple syrup, 100% pure

- a dash cayenne pepper

Recipe yields one 10 oz serving. Drink the mixture anytime through the day, up to 12 glasses daily.

Here are **some tips if you decide that this is the diet for you**:

- If you are prone to hypoglycemia, Master Cleanse is not recommended due to its high sugar levels.

- The night before you plan to start this fast, drink one cup of herbal laxative tea.

- Blend up enough for each day's serving before your first meal, adding the pepper and lemon fresh as you pour each drink, and plan on consuming 6-12 glasses per day.

- Plan on using lemons at room temperature. To best release the juices, roll them, applying firm pressure, back and forth across the countertop right before juicing.

- Don't worry about feeling lightheaded or dizzy. You could be consuming about 650-1300 calories per day from the syrup.

- Drink one cup of herbal laxative tea every evening during your fast.

- After using the Master Cleanse for 10 days, take 3 days for a successful transition back to solid foods. On Day 1, drink several glasses of orange juice throughout the day. On Day 2, eat fresh fruit and drink orange juice and vegetable broth. On Day 3, include fresh vegetables with Day 2's list of food and drinks. Return to a normal diet on the following day.

6. Selective Fasting

Selective fasting, sometimes known as *partial fasting*, combines liquid fasting with some solid food. It could range from a little bit to a lot based on your needs. The "selective" part comes from the limitation, or exclusion, of specified foods, not the amount of food consumed. Selective fasts can include mono-diets, such as fruit fasting, and cleansing diets.

You can even choose to combine some of these fasting techniques to fit around you!

HOW TO WATER FAST – ALL YOU NEED TO KNOW

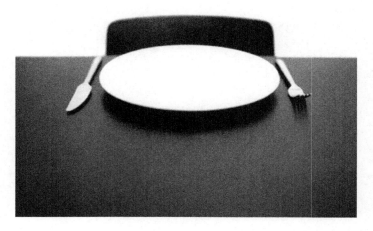

So now that you know a lot more about water fasting, it's time to look at the best ways to ensure that you fast in the most successful way for you. Here are some tips to getting it right:

What to Drink?

To do a complete water fast, you need to ensure that you consume zero calories. The most effective way to do this is by drinking water – but not just any water. You should ensure that the water you're drinking doesn't have any fluoridate or chlorinate within it. Distilled or filtered water is most recommended. This water should be warm or room temperature to get the best benefits. However you don't *only* have to drink plain water. You can add things to it to make it more interesting – lime, lemon, sea salt, and herbal teas to name just a few. (Just remember to check the amount of calories before adding these items – if it's only a few, then that's fine).

How Long?

This is entirely dependent on *you*. It's advisable to do a 24-hour fast to see how your body reacts to begin with, but the most common length of time for water fasting is between 3 and 7 days.

Is it Right for Me?

Only you can decide if water fasting is right for you. Do you have the willpower to do it? Can you clear your schedule so you can rest and distract yourself as needed? It will be difficult, so you need to be willing to put in the hard work. However, there are some people who shouldn't do it at all. This includes the very young, the very old, pregnant or breastfeeding women, and those with certain medical conditions – if you're concerned, speak to a doctor before starting.

What Exercises?

Although rest is important, so is getting exercise as you fast – particularly for the longer duration fasts. It's advisable to do none in the first week of fasting, but after that, it's good to introduce the following into your routine to make you feel much better:

- Walking
- Jogging
- Swimming
- Light cardio

Phases of Water Fasting

Your body will go through some phases as you fast. Being aware of these will make your fast much more bearable.

- **Preparation** – it's best to go on a pre-fast diet, slowly eliminate all greasy foods, meat, cigarettes, dairy products, alcohol, fish, sugar, eggs, coffee, and black tea, etc. Ensure that you're only consuming raw foods a few days before your fast.

- **Hunger** – this is more of a psychological reaction and is usually an intense desire to eat food. After three to four days of not consuming food, this 'psychological hunger' will pass. Be prepared for it, and don't lose any resolve.

- **Acidosis** – the typical Western diet includes a high proportion of acid-forming foods. After transitioning to burning fat for fuel, even more acidic substances are released in the body. It is possible for dizziness, fatigue, and blurred vision to accompany acidosis. Your urine may be concentrated and foul, your breath may smell bad, and your tongue may be coated with a bad-tasting mucus. This will pass.

- **Normalization** – most fasters will ease into the process by the end of those first seven to ten days. This is typically when the acidic blood chemistry levels out.

- **Recovery** – once the blood chemistry stabilizes, recovery can proceed swiftly. The vital force is then directed toward repair and re-generation. You may even start to feel injuries that you had forgotten all about as your body starts to fix them.

- **Breaking** – ending the fast requires just as much thought and planning as starting it. Immediately after breaking the fast, when you attempt eating solid food, your body might reject it. Digestion may be difficult, making you feel even worse. To combat this, you could ease back into solid food with a juice diet, consuming as little as possible. Start by sipping slowly, staying on juice until your digestion improves. This is when you could try small pieces of solid raw food. Diluted, raw fruit juices should be your introductory meals.

As you can see from this, the key to successful fasting is preparation. If you are educated in what will happen to you, and you know what to do when it does, then you will be much stronger mentally to see it through.

Research-Backed Guide To Lose 40 Pounds In 30 Days

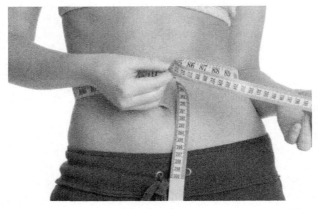

Because you are consuming zero calories during your water fast, of course, you will lose weight. It's reported that you will actually lose approximately 20 pounds in the first week of fasting, then 3 pounds per day after that, when you're performing a water fast. This style of weight loss is only really applicable if you are overweight or obese, so be sure to consult a health practitioner before you begin to check that you qualify.

Here is **what will happen to your body in the 30 days you're fasting**:

Stage 1: Days 1-2

- On the first day, your blood sugar level drops below 70mg/dl.
- The rate of internal chemical activity in resting tissue is dropped to conserve energy.
- Blood pressure drops and your heart rate slows.
- Glycogen being pulled from muscles causes some weakness.
- The first stage of detoxification includes a heavily coated tongue, headaches, bad breath, nausea, glazed eyes, and dizziness. Hunger may be its most intense during this stage.

Stage 2: Days 3-7

- Transformed fatty acids break down and discharge glycerol from glyceride molecules, then turn to glucose.

THE WATER FASTING GUIDE

- As fetid oils are removed, your skin may become oily. A pale complexion is another sign of waste in the blood.

- Ketones are formed with the incomplete oxidation of fats. For the first few days, the hunger you may feel is temporary.

- Your body begins to accept the fasting, so the digestive system will lose the body's focus, where all of that energy will be directed to cleansing organs and repairing lungs. Expect to excrete a yellow-colored mucus.

- While your colon is being repaired, impacted feces will start to loosen from the intestinal wall and get autolyzed.

Stage 3: Days 8-15

- Approaching the final half of an extended fast, you feel better than you have since youth, your energy can feel enhanced, and your mind clearer.

- However, old injuries can irritate and become painful again. This is due to the body's intensified healing ability while you're fasting.

Stage 4: Days 16-30

- Your body has completely adapted to the fasting process.

- Your lymphatic system has been cleaned, and your homeostatic balance has reached ideal levels. You may experience the rare mucus discharge from the throat or nose.

- Beyond the 20th day, your mind can experience emotional balance and mental clarity. Concentration and memory are enhanced.

Stage 5: Post-fast, beyond day 30

- Your breath turns sweet and clean, after being bad during the fast, and the bad taste that lingered in your mouth disappears.

- Your tongue is clear of the thick coating that remained through the fast.

- Your temperature returns to normal and stays, while it may have been sub-normal or above normal during the fast.

- Your pulse returns to its normal rhythm.

- Your skin and other bodily reactions return to normal.

- Your salivary secretion returns to normal.

- Your eye sight improves, and your eyes appear brighter.

- You lose the odor of excreta, and your urine becomes light.

A 30-day fast is a very long fast, so it must not be completed by beginners. It may even be advisable to do it under the supervision of health professionals. If you do choose to do it at home, here are **some tips to help you out**:

- Speak to your doctor beforehand – this is essential to ensure you get the right advice.

- Research and plan – the better prepared you are, the more successful your fast will be.

- Practice. Try out some shorter fasts to see how your body copes.

- Rest for the first week of fasting, then start to introduce some light exercise to help you along.

- Think about the side effects – it might be easier to clear your schedule and take time off work to complete your fast.

- Eat sensibly after you have completed your fast to keep the weight off. (Look at the "Breaking Your Fast" chapter for more information on this.)

So how do you go about fasting for 30 days? Obviously, this is a much longer fast, so you will need to be careful with what you do before and after your fast.

It is suggested that you complete the **cleansing diet** for 7 to 14 days before beginning the fast.

This means **banning the following from your diet**:

- Salt

- Sugar

- Fried foods

- Cheese

- Junk food of any kind

- Dairy

- Red meat

- Alcohol

THE WATER FASTING GUIDE

- Butter or Margarine
- Fruit juice
- White bread

Foods to **limit for Cleansing Diet:**

- Olive oil
- Corn or Peas
- Tomatoes
- Fruits (except for strawberries or cantaloupe)

Cleansing Diet Sample Menu

Meal 1

- 1 cup of green tea – Green tea has properties that boost energy, ease hunger, and warm your body. Sparkling or seltzer water and club soda, like green tea, can fight hunger.

- 1 cup of oatmeal with plums or raisins (suggested: 1 handful).

- 3 egg whites with ground turkey (suggested: 3 oz).

Snack 1

- 1 whole fruit (suggested: apple, banana, or pear) or 1 whole fruit (suggested: pear or apple) with 1 cup of plain, low-fat yogurt.

Meal 2

- Lettuce salad including tomato and preferred vegetables. Dressing can consist of olive oil (suggested: 1 tsp or less) or balsamic vinegar.

- 1 2.6 oz pouch of tuna (low sodium).

- 1 baked sweet potato or potato (suggested: 4 oz).

Snack 2

- Similar to Snack 1 – 1 piece of fruit (could also include yogurt), plus 1 cup of green tea.

Meal 3

- 1 serving of ground turkey, chicken, or fish (suggested: 6 oz). Salad similar to Meal 2.

- Steamed vegetables (suggested: carrots, broccoli, and cauliflower).

- Baked sweet potato or potato, brown rice, or whole wheat or whole grain pasta (suggested: 4 oz).

Snack 3

- No carbohydrates – Salad with fish, chicken, or ground turkey (suggested: 3 oz).

- 1 piece of fruit with plain, non-fat yogurt.

- 1 cup of chamomile tea – Chamomile is great to drink at night. It can promote calm, soothe hunger, and improves sleep.

THE WATER FASTING GUIDE

- After the last daily meal, water fast until you eat the first meal of the following day. This will help your body get ready for the fast, as many of your cravings will already have been dealt with.

You will then need to consider **breaking your fast** – another aspect that you need to consider very carefully, because you have been so long without food. Everything will need to be reintroduced carefully and slowly. Here are some tips to help you on this:

- Begin with 50% water, 50% fruit juice – one 8-ounce glass every four hours for the first day.

- Days 2 and 3 must be the same, just with a 12-ounce glass.

- On days 4 and 5, your digestive system will be a little more awake, so every four hours, eat a piece of fruit very slowly and then drink a 50/50 juice and water combo.

- On day 6, you can eat salads and raw vegetables. Just chew slowly and listen to what your body is telling you.

- On day 7 and after, you can start to introduce small elements of poultry. Then very slowly begin to bring back small amounts of carbohydrates to your diet.

The fast should have given you a clearer indication of your body's requests, so you should be able to know what you want and need. Just be careful and eat slowly, so that you don't make yourself ill. Continue to drink a lot, and if possible, avoid the foods listed above in the pre-fast list. Particularly junk food, fried foods, and sugar.

You *can* lose 40 pounds in 30 days with water fasting if you are prepared. This is definitely more of a lifestyle change rather than a diet, so keep that in mind at all times. Abstaining from food for this extended period of time won't be easy. You *will* need willpower, so being aware of the potential negative things that you may experience will make them much less of a shock if they appear.

If you're looking for inspiration, check out Elicia Miller on YouTube, who completed a 30-day fast and explains all of the benefits that she received from it in her blog.

34

CASE STUDIES

It's always interesting to read the case studies of people who have successfully completed a water fast, so here are some examples from the **Natural Hygiene Society** at *naturalhygienesociety.org* to give you inspiration for your own journey:

Tim

"My 49-day supervised fast (31 days on pure water; 18 on restricted coconut water and pure water)

I am writing this so that anyone considering a long fast (or indeed a short one) might have some idea of the wonders and difficulties ahead. If you read nothing else, remember this: do it; you won't regret it!

I had previously undertaken a couple of short fasts on my own. They had shown me how effective fasting can be in regaining perfect health. But intuitively I knew that I wanted to do a long fast, all the way until my hunger returned, as described in all the classic literature on fasting. I selected Maya's heavenly place in Hawai'i by sheer caprice – I liked her brilliant smile in her photograph on her website. I was so certain that I booked a 90 day stay in advance – the most the US visa people would allow me on short notice.

I was impressed with beautiful Hawai'i, the magical rural retreat center and the high-quality accommodation, and I knew straight away on meeting Maya that she was up to the task. Within a few hours of getting off the plane I was basking in hot ponds, crashing ocean surf in the background, fish nibbling at my toes and turtles swimming with us in the crystal aquamarine waters.

I had been on juices for about four days before flying, and had more or less been fasting on the airline, so pretty quickly my fast was underway full force.

There is no real way to describe a fast. Herman Hesse said that the lives of men of action are interesting to relate, but dull to live, while the lives of wasters, idlers and dreamers make terribly drab reading, but for their owners are brimming with unparalleled experiences of inspiration, hope and beauty. Fasting is just like that. Each day was so amaz-

ingly different from the previous, so stock full of wonders, but each, in essence, consisted of lying down, drinking water, going to the toilet and sleeping.

I won't relate exactly what happened to me. Nothing that I expected to happen, happened; the things I least expected to happen, did. If you hear my stories, you might expect the same things to happen to you. I can tell you of my tongue's coat changing and parting like the red sea, moles falling off, grey hairs vanishing, warts disappearing, knees and entire leg bones straightening, eyesight going wild then improving, a little toenail appearing for the first time in my life, but I can also tell you of a cyst in my nose remaining, a scar on my cheek unchanged. Who knows what your body will consider its priorities? (And who knows what miracles occurred in my kidneys, my spleen, my prostate, etc., etc.? After all, the body has a lot of nooks and crannies, and it's clever enough to repair them all, perfectly, in turn and in concert, in a conscious-numbingly fine-tuned web of co-ordinated steps and actions.)

Generally though, I am amazed at the overall rejuvenation that has occurred. My hair and eyes are shining. My brain feels like it is being fed properly (for the first time) — in essence, I am substantially cleverer. I am calmer. I am happier. I am wiser. My skin is as taught as rubber. I sat next to a super-handsome 19-year-old Olympic triathlete in the plane home and the stewardess asked if we were brothers as "we looked so alike". (I just had to tell you that.)

I haven't gone into some of the "trials" I went through - not hunger, more mental tribulations, and emotionally suffering. All I can say is that Maya was there, warm and consummately professional, and that I wouldn't change a moment of it.

All I can say is: take action, anything is possible."

Madelyn Krystal Hill

Ulcerative Colitis: A Story Of Healing

"I was 22 years old when I noticed blood in my stool. I chose to ignore it. But when it continued to recur, I came out of my denial and paid a visit to the family doctor. He diagnosed me with ulcerative colitis. My first question was: "What is causing this?" My doctor told me the cause was unknown—it could be a gene, allergy, nerves and so on. This perplexed me. No one in my family had the condition, I had no allergies, and I wasn't nervous. My next question was: "What cures it?" And he couldn't tell me the answer to that either. I proceeded to see a series of gastroenterologists, right up to the doctor who "wrote the book" and started "the foundation" in the hope that someone could cure me. Throughout this journey, I was; in and out of hospitals, took a series of invasive tests; and lived on rectal and oral medications, including sulfur and cortisone which did not agree with me. I had swelling, nightmares, difficulty concentrating, and felt disturbed much of the time. My condition worsened with time and there were days when I was so weak, in so much pain and losing so much blood that I could not get out of bed. I was told that I would soon need a colostomy and that the severity of my condition would no doubt lead to colon cancer.

After three years of severe debility which propelled me into a state of depression, I awoke one morning with an intuitive prodding and a sense of urgency to seek a new path. I instinctively knew I was doing something to contribute to my condition but didn't know what it was. I was determined to Find Out which changes I needed to make to get well. With the help of what must have been an angel, I made my way to the library and a used bookstore to research my condition. Searching for answers in many books, I found Fit Far Life by Harvey and Marilyn Diamond. When I read eat only fresh fruit till noon, I thought: "What kind of gimmick is this?" After all, I grew up in a family where we were taught to be grateful for all the food we had on the table. No one thought about whether it came from a can or ajar. I thought anyone who wouldn't eat my grandma's lamb stew (e.g. a vegetarian) was a total weirdo. But something about the book captured me, and it was from this book that I learned about Natural Hygiene, a discipline which changed my life. Natural Hygiene is not taught to doctors in medical school or influenced by government or industry. It is solely based upon biology and the immutable laws of nature which do not violate the innate wisdom of the body. I immediately elected to study it.

It was by following the tenets of Natural Hygiene, including a natural hygienic dietary, that I established the conditions for my body to heal itself. Once I learned how my choices were destroying my health (acts which I had previously not known were unhealthful), it was easy to make the changes and jump-start the innate healing powers of my body. I started out by giving up artificial sweeteners, then foods with chemicals and preservatives. I saw a remarkable improvement in my condition. Then I followed the principles of food combining and gave tip hard-to-digest combination, like yogurt with nut, and raisins. I added more and more fruits and vegetables and live foods to my diet ... and so on. Within three months, I was totally healed and haven't had a recurrence since. That was over 15 years ago.

Today, it is estimated that approximately 30,000 women each year die from colon cancer, the third most common cancer among women in the United States. Health care costs are soaring, yet there are no "cures." I am sharing my story with you in the hope that more and more patients and clinicians will seek out systemic truths and open their eyes and ears to the tenets of Natural Hygiene in determining both the cause of disease and principles of healing.

Don't ever let anyone take away your hope. Especially you."

Dr. Dimitri Karalis

My first water fast in 1972

"There is no better way for a diseased and prematurely aged body to be restored back to robust health, than through the fasting vehicle. A complete supervised fasting by an experienced doctor is the safest, quickest and surest way to health, beauty, and happiness for all mental and physical sufferers. It restores not only the precious health, but also opens new horizons for mental and spiritual possibilities that were never dreamed of before. A new lease of life derives from it, like being reborn again in life. Body, mind and soul become so serene and harmonious together, that one feels so peaceful and confident as if sitting in the lap of God. No matter how sick you are or what your life problems are, nature wants always to assist you if you give her a chance. A supervised fast is the only way that can bring all your heart desires if you persist with it wisely to the end. Health, beauty, power, success, courage, freedom, peace, inspiration, spirituality and love, all are yours after a successful fast.*

When I took my first water fast in 1972, I had the most amazing pleasant experience one night. I woke at midnight on the 17th day of my fasting, feeling buoyant and with a strong desire for running. I tried to reason for a while by ignoring this strange midnight longing and to go back to sleep. Yet my love for it was so overpowering that I went running instead at one o'clock in the morning. After four hours of running, I lost all my gravity and I felt as if I was weightless with a total lack of fatigue. All of nature around me took on a wonderful hue and I felt so eager to greet every human being who passed me by. I felt exceptionally happy and my only wish was how to express and transmit this wonderful feeling that I was experiencing to others. I discovered at the same time, that love and happiness is a product of perfect health, of harmonious functioning body, mind and soul. Nothing else can give it to us, except a perfect functioning metabolism like in the healthy infant.

All negative habits like fear, doubts, jealousy, envy, hate and lack of confidant, disappear after a long successful fast. You can easily say that one has been reborn again like a baby. Why don't you give this natural and absolute safe method the chance to help you? What do you lose by cleaning the blood, body, skin, mind, and soul and renewing your inner organs again? Are the lethal drugs with the vandalizing surgical knives more attractive to you? Why don't you trust the fasting instinct method as all the animals do when they are sick? Whatever your physical and mental problems are at the moment, there is definitely a better solution for you than pain, depression, worry and sorrow every day. Try to find a qualified and well experience doctor in your area, and obey to his fasting instruction. Not only you will achieve better health with proper fasting, but you will also open new outlook in life with a happier and brighter future that you never dreamed of before."

And here is an example of **what someone went through on their 10-day fast**, from ***Don't Waste the Crumbs*** (*dontwastethecrumbs.com*):

"Days 1-3. The first few days were rough. It was during this time that the detoxifying symptoms were the worst. There was hunger, splitting headaches… it was rough. I am a coffee lover (as most parents are). Nothing beats pouring a hot cup of freshly brewed coffee into a ceramic mug, sipping the java goodness before starting the day. I attribute the pure misery of days 1-3 to caffeine withdrawal. At the same time, Mrs. Crumbs cooking dinner for the kids and knowing I couldn't eat was brutal.

Days 4-6. These days were relatively easy. By this time my digestive system had shut down and the hunger pains had disappeared. My tongue was often coated with a thick white film. This is apparently normal and another detoxification symptom. I started losing weight – 1 – ½ pounds per day – but there was no problem going to work, playing guitar at church or performing any other daily physical functions.

Day 7. I will never forget this day – ever. This was the most miserable day I have ever lived on planet earth. I came home from work feeling great, not hungry, thinking clearly… And then my life was flipped upside down. My wonderful wife pulled a freshly baked loaf of rosemary bread from the oven. I was immediately angry and I wanted that bread. But it wasn't even possible at this point.

You see, once your digestive system shuts down (around the three-day mark), it takes a few days to bring it back up to speed. You do this by very slowly introducing food to your digestive system… drinking juice for 1-2 days, fresh fruit for another couple days, steamed vegetables for another day or two… taking anywhere from 7 – 14 days to bring your digestive system back up to fully operational. Eating any solid food while in a fasted state can lead to severe discomfort and even hospitalization!

Back to the bread… I wanted that bread so much that I had to go upstairs, take a shower and wait for everyone to finish eating dinner. I simply could not bear even LOOKING at the bread!

Day 8-10. These days were almost an exact replica of days 4-6. By the end of day 10, I had lost 15 pounds and was ready to eat again."

So as you have seen, there are difficulties with water fasting – your mental strength is very likely to be tested – but the possible rewards that you can receive at the end of your water fast will make it all worth it!

5 SAFETY TIPS YOU WISH YOU KNEW

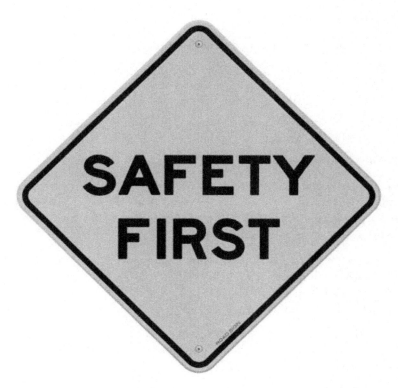

There are some **safety tips** that you should be aware of before starting a water fast. These will ensure that you do this in the healthiest way possible.

1. Check that you *can* fast before starting.

It's important to be aware that there are **groups of people that *shouldn't***

fast. This includes:

- Children
- Elderly people
- Women who are pregnant or breastfeeding
- Those with insufficient kidney function
- People who suffer from diabetes

If you suffer from any medical condition, or you take medications, you should consult a doctor before starting your fast.

2. Consider doing a supervised fast.

There are some situations where **doing a water fast under the supervision of health professionals** is advisable. This includes:

- Fasting for an extended period of time.
- If you're doing the fast to alleviate serious diseases.
- If you're extremely overweight.
- If you suffer from any emotional problems – because emotions often become entangled in food.

3. Know when to break the fast.

Breaking the fast at the right time is essential for you to remain healthy and maintain the results that you have received from fasting. There are certain things to look out for, and even if you've planned to fast for longer, **these are signs that you should end it** now:

- *Low potassium levels* – symptoms include: irritability and mental confusion, fatigue, irregular heartbeat; muscle weakness, fatigue, and cramps. This means you need to drink some juice and begin breaking the fast right away.

- *A taste of heavy metals* – if you experience this in your mouth, it may not be a good idea to continue with water. This could mean heavy metals are being flushed from your body.

- *Physical cleansing reactions* – normal fasting side effects include blurred vision, headaches, minor aches and pains, fatigue, nausea, heartburn and acid reflux, skin rashes or eruptions, and trouble sleeping. These are normal, but if the reactions become extreme, you will need to break your fast.

THE WATER FASTING GUIDE

- *Emotional cleansing reactions* – you will likely experience some negative emotions such as anger, guilt, sadness, and depression. These emotions typically manifest when the liver is being cleansed, so see these emotions as a good sign. Your body is releasing these deep-rooted energies from its cells once and for all.

- *Hunger* – this is the side effect that most people predominantly worry about. The more you think about food and the more you're around it, the hungrier you will feel. However, if your body goes into 'starvation mode' for too long, you will start to feel really ill. If this happens, it's time to break the fast.

This topic is covered in more detail in a later chapter of this book.

4. Prepare well.

The absolute best tip for fasting is preparation. The more that you are ready for it, the more successful your fast will be. There is a chapter covering this in more detail later in this book, but here are some key points to remember for now:

- *Clear your schedule* – there may be times where you need to rest and there may be times when you need to keep yourself busy and distracted. A clear schedule will allow you to do what's necessary.

- *Have everything to hand* – go shopping before you start your fast to ensure that you have all of your supplements and teas, etc. before getting started.

- *Educate yourself* – find out everything you need to know about fasting before you begin. The more you know, the more successful your fast will be.

- *Eat smaller meals* – on the days leading up to your fast, eat less to help prepare your body.

- *Connect with others* – use online forums and local groups to speak to others who are going through the same thing. Sometimes the best advice can come from people who have done a fast before.

- *Speak to your doctor* – get personalized advice about your water fast before starting.

On top of this, prepare yourself mentally for what you're about to do. The stronger your mind is, the more powerful your willpower will be.

5. Be aware of the side effects of water fasting.

If you're aware of what you might experience, then you will be more equipped to deal with these side effects if they come along. The most common side effects of fasting are trouble sleeping, fatigue, headaches, nausea, skin rashes or eruptions, minor aches and pains, heartburn and acid reflux, and blurred vision.

MOST COMMON MISTAKES AND HOW TO AVOID THEM

There are some mistakes that people make when water fasting, and avoiding these will ensure that you're much more successful in reaching your end goals.

- Giving up too quickly. You *need* to give yourself time to adjust. It *will* be difficult at times; you just need the mental strength to overcome that.

- Doing it too quickly. You need to decrease your meal sizes over time before your fast, to allow your stomach to shrink in preparation.

- Fasting for too long. When the signs that you should break your fast start to appear, pay attention to your body and do it. Otherwise you risk making yourself unnecessarily unwell.

- Not drinking enough water. This is very important. Your body will need to get enough water to get through this. Sip it throughout the day.

- Expecting too much. You *will* get benefits from doing this, just don't expect too much too soon.

- Smoking and drinking alcohol while water fasting makes it much harder to stick to as they have negative side effects on the body.

- Telling others what you're doing can be negative as they will offer 'helpful' opinions, which actually put you off the fast.

- Being too hard on yourself – if you slip up, don't make it the be all and end all. Pick yourself up, dust yourself off, and try again.

The important thing to remember is that you probably *will* make some mistakes, despite your best intentions not to. As long as you get back on track, the error can be something that you learn from, rather than the thing that derails you. Here are some great **tips for overcoming these obstacles**, and staying motivated:

- Keep your end goal at the forefront of your mind. You're doing this for a reason, something about it is important to you. Don't let yourself forget that.

- Keep positive. You *will* eat again. Don't allow yourself to sink into the bad moods that come your way.

- Keep busy and distracted and avoid needless temptation. Being around food makes it a lot harder to avoid.

- Rest if you need to rest! Don't allow fatigue or dizziness to consume you. Your body will let you know when it needs to rest, so listen to it.

- Speak to your doctor if you're at all worried – sometimes just to get confirmation that you're doing okay and you're staying healthy is enough to keep you going.

- Have someone to talk to – a friend, a family member, even the online forums. Having someone to keep you going when things are tough might be all that you need.

- Keep motivational quotes posted around your home and on your fridge. Read them when you need encouragement!

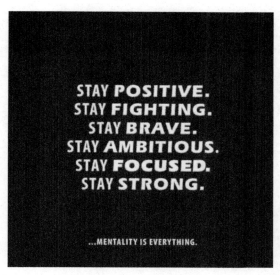

It is suggested that **if negative feelings and emotions *do* come up during your fast**, then you will need to the following:

- **Identify which emotions you're feeling**. There will be times when different emotions could hit you all at once. Try to identify as many as possible, then pick just one to focus on. After you have achieved closure with that emotion, you can move on to the others.

- **Try to understand where these emotions stem from**. After you identify the emotion, ask why you're feeling it. Some of your answers may be: "I'm depressed" or "Because life is hard," but these answers are only on the first level. Explore your answers more deeply by analyzing them. You could get answers that link back to past life events if you do this with time and patience.

- As you achieve that awareness, **think about exactly how that event is connected to that emotion**. If you see events as unbiased situations, then our interpretations of those situations become independent of those events and we can begin to understand how we tie emotions to events. You can achieve closure, figure out a conclusion, once you have successfully analyzed how that emotion occurred.

Since most of your fasting obstacles will likely be in your mind, this process should help you maintain control of your emotional responses.

You will need to remain strong throughout the fast. Speaking to a health professional can help you with this.

8 INSIDER TIPS
TO STARTING A FAST

The way that you prepare for a water fast will determine how successful you are. **Here are some tips for ensuring that you are fully ready for your own fast**:

1. Speak to your doctor.

This is the most important thing for you to do. You need to consult a health professional to check that you're eligible to fast, that it's the right move for you, and you can also get some personalized advice, tailored just for you.

2. Set your goals and work out all of the fasting details accordingly.

The first thing you need to do is decide why you're doing your fast. Is it for weight loss? The health benefits? Something else? Whatever it is, setting a specific, defined goal will give you something to aim for – helping to keep you motivated.

When looking at your goals, it's always advisable to be **SMART**:

- Set a **S**pecific goal
- Choose **M**easurable objectives
- Make sure goals/objectives are **A**chievable
- Establish **R**easonable parameters
- Set up goals/objectives that are **T**ime-based

An example of creating a SMART goal for your fast would look like this:

'I want to do a water fast because of the health benefits that it offers.'

- **Specific** – You will need to make this more specific. 'I will start with a 24-hour fast to see how my body reacts.'

- **Measurable** – What measurable objectives will you set to ensure that you keep up with this? 'I will set aside two weeks to do this towards the end of the month.'

- **Achievable** – Is this possible? 'I will prepare myself for this fast for a week beforehand. I will break the fast slowly, over a week.'

- **Reasonable** – Are you really going to be able to do this? 'I will see how I feel once the fast has been broken, then re-evaluate.'

- **Time-based** – You will want to keep an eye on your progress, to check that you're heading towards your goal. 'I will experiment with this 24-hour fast, then move on to 3-day fasts.'

Setting goals in this way has proven benefits and will help you meet them. They are much more structured, clearly possible, and leave nothing to hold you back.

3. Get organized and set yourself a suitable schedule.

Being fully prepared and writing out a schedule will help you keep your goal clear ahead of you when you're fasting. You'll need to consider:

- Time to rest if necessary and time to keep busy and distracted – clearing your schedule will allow you to do whatever's necessary at the time for you.

- Shopping – get everything ready, have everything that you're going to need in the cupboard before you start your fast.

- Help – you might need it along the way. Whether this is from your doctor, others going through the same as you, or your friends and family, having someone there will help keep you motivated.

Organization is key to completing a successful fast. The better prepared that you are, the more likely you'll be to do this!

4. Prepare your mindset.

Your mind will become your biggest supporter – or your largest critic – when water fasting. Getting into the right mindset will ensure that you are successful. Meditation can actually help you with this, as it helps you live in the present moment, distracting yourself and taking away any stress, easing you into the fast.

Meditation might seem like an odd partner for fasting, but it has proven benefits that *will* help you. Try these **six simple mindfulness exercises** to get you started:

Focused Breathing

This exercise is very easy and can be performed anywhere, from any position, and at any time during the day or night. You only need to focus on the act of breathing and stay still for just one minute.

- Start by slowly breathing in and out, focusing on the air entering then leaving your body. Inhale through your nose; exhale through your mouth. One deep breath will last about 6 seconds.

- Clear your thoughts for 1 minute. Dismiss thoughts about household chores, pending projects, or things stuck on your to-do list. Allow yourself to be still for just 1 minute.

- Monitor your breath, focus on your senses by feeling, hearing each breath as it fills your body – infuses you with life. Feel its energy work its way up from your lungs, then out of your mouth as it dissipates into the world.

Try two or three minutes of this centering exercise if you've enjoyed the one-minute version described above.

> " Mindfulness means paying attention in a particular way; On purpose, in the present moment, and non-judgmentally. "
>
> Jon Kabat-Zinn

Focused Observation

This simple, yet powerful exercise is used to connect our minds with the environment's natural beauty. Something like that is often missed while we are bustling through the day's planned and unexpected events.

- Select one natural object that you can see clearly from where you are sitting. Focus on it just a minute or two. Good examples are a flower, an insect, the clouds, or the moon.

- Look at your selected object as if you are seeing it for the first time. Clear your mind of anything else, only focus on the object. Take more than a minute or two if needed; sit and concentrate until you relax into mental harmony.

- Examine each aspect of this object. Be consumed by your focus. Concentrate on this object's energy as well as its purpose and role in the world.

Focused Awareness

Similar to the exercise of focusing on an object, Focused Awareness encourages you to apply heightened attention toward the results of common daily tasks.

- Bring to mind an activity or task that occurs daily, more than once; something you might take for granted, such as, opening a window. The moment you touch the frame to slide it open, be aware of how you feel, where you stand, and what the window looks out toward. Or, as another example, apply Focused Awareness when you open your laptop to work. Take just a moment, or more, if needed, and concentrate on your brain facilitating the understanding to use this machine and how your hands work to open it.

- The moments and acts we mentioned are called touch points, and those suggestions can be touch points other than the physical ones. For example, whenever you experience a degrading thought you could take a moment to stop, identify the thought as powerless, and then let that negativity go. Another example is focusing on the moment when you cook food. Make it a point to stop and concentrate on your luck at having good food to eat, knowing how to prepare it, being able to prepare it, and being able to eat it.

This exercise works better when you choose a touch point that resonates with you. Select occasional moments where you can stop and concentrate on the actions you take rather than going through those daily motions on autopilot. Cultivating this Focused Awareness for the blessings that exist in your life will improve and strengthen your mindset.

Focused Listening

This exercise is designed to teach you to open your ears to sounds without judgment. Many sounds we hear every day are influenced by past events, however, if we make the effort to focus when we listen, we can achieve this neutral, present awareness where we consume sounds without prejudice.

- Choose a piece of music you have never listened to before, either from a personal music collection or by scanning local radio stations.

- Use your headphones, then close your eyes so you won't see the song's title, genre, or artist name. While the song plays, dismiss thoughts about labels and get lost in the sound of the music. Explore every element of the song. Especially if it isn't a song that you would normally listen to, dismiss your initial reaction and allow your perception to fully explore the song and enjoy the sound simply for what it is.

Your goal is to focus your listening and get fully immersed with the song after intentionally dismissing judgment or prejudice for the genre, lyrics, instrumentation, or artist.

Focused Immersion

This exercise is designed to help you find comfort in the present and avoid the feeling of constantly striving we experience every day. When you feel anxious to complete an everyday routine task, take a look at that regular routine from a different perspective and experience it in a new way.

As an example, think about how you normally feel when the garage needs to be organized. Normally, it feels like a chore and no one wants to do it. However, when you focus on every detail of the activity, you can create a pleasant experience by becoming fully immersed in each detail of your actions. Feel every muscle stretch when you move boxes, truly experience the motion as you sweep up the floor, watch your hands wipe away dust and cobwebs, admire the color of the fluid you spray to clean the windows. Your goal is to discover fresh experiences while performing a routine chore.

When you fully immerse in the process and focus on every step, you can center yourself within every activity mentally, physically, and spiritually, and think of it as more than a boring routine.

Focused Appreciation

For this exercise, your goal is to list 5 things from your day that are typically unappreciated. This list is personalized and specific to you – the 5 things could be people or objects. Make this list of 5 before the end of your day.

There is a certain power in being able to appreciate and genuinely give thanks even for the things you might take for granted, the objects that support our existence but barely get a second thought in our pursuit for bigger and better things.

For instance: your oven is powered by electricity, your mail is regularly delivered by a friendly postman, your clothes aren't torn and provide warmth, you can play catch in the park with your kids, you can hear birds chirping in the tree outside your window, but...

- Have you ever stopped to focus on the details or finer elements of these things?

- Have you ever noticed the benefit these things bring to your life and others' lives?

- Have you ever considered correlations between these things and how they all play an interconnected role in daily life?

- Do you know how these aspects of daily life work or even how they exist?

- Have you ever wondered what life would be like without these things?

After you choose your 5 things, make it a point to learn everything that you can about their origin and purpose in order to truly acknowledge how they enhance life.

If this is something that you're interested in, and want to learn more, try out the audio led mindfulness exercises at **Living Well** from *www.livingwell.org.au.*

5. Prepare your body.

You will need to get your body ready for the fast. Here are **some tips for the days leading up to your fast**:

- A few days before your fast, reduce intake of salt, caffeine, sugar, meats, and cooked food, etc. Removing them from your diet suddenly can cause a general sense of discomfort, including stomachaches and headaches.

- Start eating smaller meals before your fast, also. Resist the very real temptation of eating a large "last supper." Eating smaller meals a few days in advance trains your stomach, appetite, and mind for your fast.

- Make it a point to eat more fresh things instead of cooked food.

- Drink mild herbal teas on the days leading up to your fast.

- Consume the fresh vegetable and fruit juices you like, especially with dark greens, before you fast.

- Eliminate sweets, eggs, refined flour products, fried foods, and dairy products from your diet before your fast.

- When cooking in the days and weeks before your fast, don't use butter, margarine, or salt.
- Drink a 'green drink,' plus a cup of ginger tea steeped with fresh, warm lemon water each day, if possible.

6. Work out your nutrition.

To ensure that you remain healthy, you will need to think about your metabolism – not only during your fast, but the rest of the time too. Supplements are a great way to ensure that you're getting anything that you are missing. Here are the most commonly used supplements when fasting. These only contain a small number of calories, so they won't affect your daily totals too drastically:

- *Branched Chain Amino Acids* – an essential nutrient that we have to get from food or supplements, because our bodies do not produce it.
- *Calcium* – increases fat excretion and boosts testosterone.
- *Vitamin D* – helps you function optimally.
- *Creatine* – helps boost muscle.
- *Beta Alanine* – boosts exercise performance.
- *Glucosamine* – ideal for relieving joint pain.

7. Sort out your pre-fast routine.

Getting this part of the fast right is essential to your chances of success. Here is a Pre-Fast Regimen that accounts for eight days of **fast preparation**:

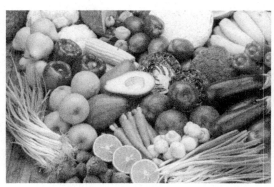

- *Days 1, 2, 3*: Avoid legumes, meat, eggs fowl, fish dairy, spices and salt, and grains. Fruits and vegetables are acceptable; feel free to cook them.

- *Days 4, 5, 6*: Continue regimen from first three days, except fruits and vegetables should be eaten raw.

- *Days 7 and 8*: Consume only vegetable juices and raw fruit.

Here are some **tips for choosing the right food before you fast**:

- Teach yourself to read labels – this information helps you know the ingredients of the food you are eating.

- Eat raw fruits and vegetables as often as you can handle (most people follow a 60% raw and 40% cooked proportion). If you have weak digestion, try eating baked or steamed vegetables and then take digestive enzyme supplements.

- Before you start the cleanse, consume raw, organic vegetable juices per day, and there is no limit on how much you can drink. In fact, the more you drink, the less hunger you will feel, and you'll be giving your body nutrition, as well as hindering cravings.

- The following recipes are great for raw, organic pre-fast smoothies:
  - Blend: 2 cups of water, 2 celery sticks, 1/2 red onion, 1/2 lime (juiced), 6 leaves of red leaf lettuce, 1/4 bunch of fresh basil, and 1/4 avocado.
  - Blend: 2 cups of water, 3 cloves garlic, 1/2 lime (juiced), 5 kale leaves (green), 1/2 bunch of fresh dill, and 1/4 cup sundried tomatoes.

- Drink water as often as you can, because it is an important aspect of the fasting process. Try to drink approximately 6% of your current body weight (i.e. 65 kg body weight, drink 3.9 liters of water) on a warmer day, and 3% will suffice on a cooler day. This only applies to water, not other drinks such as fruit juice, tea, or coffee.

- Restrict snacking to fruits, vegetable juices, mineral/vegetable broths.

- Post-fast, your goal will be eating less food, and if you start doing that beforehand, that preparation will make the fasting process easier on your body and mind.

Here are is a **sample pre-fast diet** lasting for a week before starting your fast:

Allowed Foods for this Diet:

THE WATER FASTING GUIDE

- *Vegetables* – Turnips, Artichokes, Radishes, Asparagus, Peppers, Aubergine, Parsley, Beans, Onions, Beetroot, Mushrooms, Broccoli, Lettuce, Brussels Sprouts, Sorrel, Cabbage, Chicory, Carrots, Endive, Cauliflower, Spinach, Celery, Cucumber, and Courgettes.

- *Fruits* – Tangerines, Apples, Strawberries, Apricots, Plums, Berries, Pineapple, Blueberries, Peaches, Cherries, Oranges, Grapefruit, Nectarines, Grapes, Melons, Kiwi Fruit, and Lemons. (You can consume a select number of tomatoes on day 5, and as many as you like on day 6.)

- *Food flavorings* – You are allowed nearly any no- or low-calorie flavoring of your choice, including lemon juice, dried or fresh herbs, ketchup, hot sauces, vinegars, and soy sauce. If you need something sweet, choose a low-calorie sweetener rather than sugar.

Sample Menu:

Day 1

- 1 pint cabbage soup (recipe yields about 12 pints)

  - 1 cabbage

  - 6 carrots

  - 6 medium onions

  - 6 spring onions

  - 2 red or green bell peppers, de-seeded

  - 3 tomatoes, large

  - 5 celery stalks, trimmed

  - 110g (approximately 1/2 cup) brown rice, uncooked

  - Mince vegetables and place in the 12-pint pot. Cover vegetables with cold water; bring to a boil. Simmer for almost 10 minutes, uncovered. Then simmer, covered, over low heat about an hour or until vegetables are soft. While the stock simmers, prepare rice following packet instructions. Add rice when soup is almost cooked. After soup has cooled, store where convenient, in the freezer or refrigerator.

- Eat raw fruit of your choice, except bananas

- Plain tea or coffee (artificial sweetener allowed), cranberry juice

Day 2

- 1 pint cabbage soup

- Any cooked, fresh, or raw vegetables you prefer. Dry beans, sweet corn, or peas are not allowed.

- Plain tea or coffee (artificial sweetener allowed), cranberry juice (unsweetened) and water, 1 tablespoon salad dressing (low- or no-fat)

Day 3

- 1 pint cabbage soup

- Eat any fruit you prefer, except bananas; eat any cooked, fresh, raw vegetables you prefer. Dry beans, sweet corn, or peas are not allowed.

- Plain tea or coffee (artificial sweetener allowed), cranberry juice (unsweetened) and water, 1 tablespoon salad dressing (low- or no-fat)

Day 4

- 1 pint cabbage soup

- Bananas, up to 6, are allowed in order to reduce your craving for sweets

Day 5

- 1 pint cabbage soup

- Up to 6 tomatoes

- Plain tea or coffee (artificial sweetener allowed), cranberry juice (unsweetened) and water, 1 tablespoon salad dressing (low- or no-fat)

- Drink at least 8 glasses of water to flush uric acid out of your system

Day 6

- 1 pint cabbage soup

- Unlimited vegetables, including tomatoes

THE WATER FASTING GUIDE

- Plain tea or coffee (artificial sweetener allowed), cranberry juice (unsweetened) and water, 1 tablespoon salad dressing (low- or no-fat)

Day 7

- 1 pint cabbage soup

- Any cooked, fresh, or raw vegetables you prefer. Dry beans, sweet corn, or peas are not allowed.

- Plain tea or coffee (artificial sweetener allowed), cranberry juice (unsweetened) and water, 1 tablespoon salad dressing (low- or no-fat)

Some people even chose to only **drink juice for the days before their water fast** – to get their bodies ready and to kick-start their detox. You can even do this after the diet listed above. If this is something you'd like to do, here is a *sample 3-day menu.*

Day #1

- *Meal 1 Juice:* Grapefruit Apple Juice

  - Core 2 apples, peel 2 grapefruits and juice them together.

- *Meal 2 Juice:* Orange Kale Lemon

  - Peel 3 oranges and juice them with 1 lemon and 1 handful of kale.

- *Snack 1 Juice:* Consume 1 glass of vegetable or fruit juice of your choice. You could blend one from your leftover fruits and vegetables.

- *Meal 3 Juice:* Apple Carrot Ginger

  - Core 2 apples and, if needed, remove the tops from 4 carrots. Juice carrots and apples with 1 small ginger knob.

- *Snack 2:* Herbal (no caffeine) tea that you prefer

Day #2

- *Meal 1 Juice:* Orange Pineapple

  - Remove rind from and core a pineapple; cut half of it into spears (keep other half for Day #3). Peel 2 oranges. Juice them together.

- *Meal 2 Juice:* Spinach Tomato Carrot
  - Cut 3 tomatoes into wedges. Juice 3 carrots and 1 small handful of spinach with tomato wedges.
- *Snack 1 Juice:* Consume 1 glass of your favorite fruit or vegetable juice.
- *Meal 3 Juice:* Carrot Apple Beet
  - Core 1 apple. Juice apple with 4 carrots and 1/2 beet.
- *Snack 2:* Herbal (no caffeine) tea

Day #3

- *Meal 1 Juice:* Apple Strawberry Carrot
  - Core 1 apple and juice with 2 carrots and 2 cups of strawberries.
- *Meal 2 Juice:* Tomato Orange Celery
  - Peel 2 oranges and juice with 1 tomato and 2 celery stalks.
- *Snack 1 Juice:* Consume 1 glass of your preferred vegetable or fruit juice.
- *Meal 3 Juice:* Pineapple Kale
  - Take the leftover 1/2 pineapple from Day #2, cut it into strips, and juice it with 5 leaves of kale.

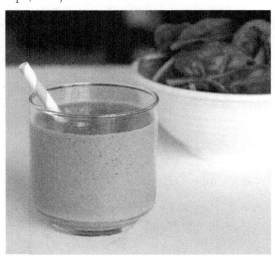

THE WATER FASTING GUIDE

8. Set your environment.

To ensure that your water fast is successful, you will need to create the right environment for yourself. Make sure that you've considered:

- Staying off work – some of the side effects are unpleasant, and there may be periods where you need to rest.

- Resting will be important during your fast, but so will distractions. Make sure that you have stuff to keep your mind occupied and off food. Take up a new hobby, reconnect with old friends, or even do some mild exercise. Just give yourself something to *do*.

- Don't tell everyone, but *do* tell someone what you're doing. Just make sure that it's someone who will encourage you and motivate you if you begin to struggle.

- Motivate yourself. Make sure that you remember *why* you're doing your water fast at all times.

As long as your environment is stress free and supportive, you will have the best chance at being successful with your fast. You don't want to start it and give up over something silly!

7 TOP TIPS FOR MANAGING YOUR FAST

You may be surprised to find that water fasting is actually easy to do, if you do it right, so here are some tips to help you get it right:

1. Consume zero calories.

Although you can't have any calories, it doesn't only have to be from water. There are other things that you can drink, including herbal teas and tea or coffee without milk. Supplements also don't count as calories and can help you get the macronutrients that your body needs.

2. Get your water right.

Getting the water right for your water fast is important. You don't want to drink tap water; you'll want to have mineral or distilled water. You will also need to drink the right amount of water. It's commonly suggested that men need to drink nearly 3 liters of water (approximately 13 cups) each day of fasting, and women need to drink nearly 2.2 liters (approximately 9 cups) each day of fasting.

Another factor that is often overlooked is the temperature of the water that you should be drinking. It is suggested that you should *only* **drink warm/room temperature water** when fasting because:

- Cold water solidifies fats in your stomach rather than dissolving them. When the fat solidifies, your body wastes energy to restore it to its original state.

- Cold water will hinder digestion because the body wastes even more energy trying to heat the water up.

- Warm/room temperature water aids detoxification. As you consume hot or warm water, your body temperature increases to enhance the detoxification process. It can stimulate sweating, which is a common way of flushing toxins from your body.

- Hot water promotes digestion and regular bowel movements by dissolving fats and food more quickly in your stomach and assisting your intestines with the movement of waste.
- Hot water enhances metabolism and the breakdown of your body's adipose tissue, which helps with weight loss.
- Hot water loosens the buildup of mucus. Expelling mucus is a way to eliminate toxins during a water fast. Warm water alleviates nasal congestion and helps clear the respiratory tract by dissolving toxins that climb into your mouth, then on your tongue, to clean the throat.
- Hot and warm water are better for clearing and hydrating your skin.

You can either pre-boil this water and let it cool to room temperature or you can buy it bottled and leave it out of the fridge – whatever suits you best.

3. Pick the right times for your water.

One of the most important things to do is drink water first thing in the morning. This will help set you up for the rest of the day. After that, the choice is yours. Some people prefer to sip water throughout the day – the only danger of this is you'll need to be sure that you've drunk enough. Others like to set out a schedule of every 2 hours or so. This is why doing a 24-hour water fast in advance is a good idea – you can figure out what the right choice for you is.

4. Look out for detox symptoms.

Knowing what is merely a detox symptom, rather than something to worry about, will help you if and when they crop up during your fast. If you're expecting them, then they won't be surprising and off-putting when they happen.

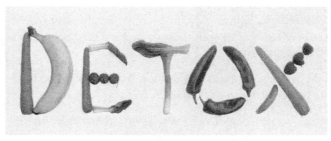

It is suggested that *"Most of these reactions are not symptoms of fasting but years of neglect, facing years of unhealthy eating manifested by pounds of unnecessary fat and toxins."* They include:

- *Hunger* – most people are surprised by how quickly the physical sensations of hunger stop showing themselves. Cravings may still be there, but your hunger will have stilled.

- *Weakness* – decreased energy is a common result of water fasting. This is a part of the slowing down process that fasting gives you. Give yourself time to rest because of this.

- *Back Pain* – toxins in the lower intestine can increase back pain. The blood vessels that draw nutrients out of the colon are near the spinal nerves. Back pain will often be alleviated after toxins have been eliminated. This can be relieved with the use of back exercises or cold compresses.

- *Foul Breath* – waste will pass through the lungs because they are an eliminative organ. Reduce bad breath by brushing your teeth and tongue, rinsing with mouthwash, and using dental floss regularly.

- *Canker Sores* – an increase of bacteria collecting between the teeth is often caused by toxic build-up inside the mouth due to the lack of chewing food and its washing action. Waste coats your tongue. Alleviate cankers by gargling with a sea salt and water mixture several times per day. Speed up the healing process with topical application of vitamin E or tea tree oil.

- *Common Cold* – a result of the fast is dumping large quantities of toxins and mucus into the bloodstream, which can cause a susceptibility to the common cold. Keep fasting in order to eliminate mucus and fight the cold.

- *Loss of Consciousness* – the body wants to conserve energy during a fast. Your heart will pump more slowly, which will reduce blood pressure. Dizziness and blackouts could be triggered by standing up or moving too quickly from an at-rest position, causing blood to rush to your legs. Prevent a loss of consciousness by sitting down or even getting down on one knee. Dropping your center of gravity will work immediately to keep you from blacking out.

- *Tension Headaches* – toxins can cause muscle tightness in your shoulders and neck, and this can generate tension headaches. Tension can be relieved by topical massage of the area of concern.

- *Tight Muscles* – muscles can become sore, tight because of toxin irritation. Legs, specifically, may be affected because toxins can settle in their large muscles. Release these toxins by applying self-massage, exercising, hot baths, and stretching.

- *Sour Stomach* – the sensation of nausea can be caused after waste has been released by the lymph glands. Where the liver takes some of the toxic overload, which is secreted into the stomach with bile. Continue drinking water to dilute the bile and toxin mixture and flush it from your body.

- *Nervous Tension* – elimination of toxins can further damage already irritated nerves. Relieve tension with light exercise.

- *Skin Blemishes* – people who otherwise never have skin problems may experience a few days where pimples or other breakouts appear. Another signal of waste in your blood is a pale complexion. Once cleansed of toxins and mucus, the skin will appear healthier, softer, and unblemished.

- *Lethargy* – sleepiness is typical during a water fast. Very few people get enough rest as it is. So the excess sleep can prove just as rejuvenating and healing as the water fast itself.

Of course, if you notice anything that worries you, then consult your doctor – they will be able to give you the best advice for you.

5. Make your water more interesting.

You can add things to your water to make your fast much more interesting. This includes lime, sea salt, and herbal teas – anything to make you feel like you're having some variety, without consuming any calories. Here is one example to give you an idea on how to keep your water interesting while on a fast:

Watermelon Flavored Water

Ingredients:

- 2 cups watermelon (seedless), cubed

- 4 cups distilled water

Directions:

- Add watermelon to a pitcher, then cover with the water.

- Store in the refrigerator for a couple hours so the water absorbs the watermelon flavor before drinking.

6. Cleanse yourself with enemas.

An enema is an alternative therapy to help cleanse your colon and rid you of diarrhea – which is often an issue after you have broken your fast. To perform an enema, fluid is injected in the lower bowel via the rectum. Commonly, an enema is used a cleansing method administered to relieve constipation or to check diarrhea. This is something you can do with your doctor, or you can get a home kit and do it yourself if you'd prefer.

This is considered by many as an essential part of water fasting. **My Fasting** at *myfasting.com* suggests that it's a vital procedure for beginners or those completing a long-term fast.

"Cleansing bowels with the ordinary enema causes considerable decreasing all these unpleasant effects. It promotes faster excretion of fat cellular debris, empties lower bowels of impacted feces; the absorbed water quickly gets into the blood, decreases intoxication, and increases urination. As a result, the unpleasant symptoms are abated. All fasting people note this. If enemas are not used the body intoxication could be so acute that you cannot continue fasting any longer. That's why using enemas is crucial for the beginners during fasting longer than 2-3 days."

In fact, the site offers these rules when it comes to enemas and water fasting:

- Enemas are vital for beginners who are fasting for longer than 1-2 days.

- Beginners should administer enemas once or twice daily during a 7-10-day fast to prevent the negative side effects of water fasting.

- After 7-10 days, the enema can be used less. Maybe once every 2-3 days.

You will also want to consider this due to the possibility of developing a condition known as *Ascaris Intestinal Roundworm* – which is a parasitic roundworm found in your intestines that can be discovered during water fasting as your body cleanses it's system. An enema can help you with this.

It is suggested that the **signs that can indicate if you have this type of Roundworm**, include:

- Digestive problems

- Chronic diarrhea, due to poor food absorption

- Excessive bowel movements

- Chronic constipation

- Mucus in stool

- Abdominal pain

- Bloating and gas, especially after meals

- Frequent vomiting and nausea

- Leaky gut

- Burning in the stomach

- Intestinal irritation

- Hemorrhoids

- Blood in stool

- Intestinal obstruction

- Pancreatitis

- Malabsorption syndrome

- Swollen eyes

- Fever

- Fatigue – Metabolizing toxic waste overloads the eliminating organs, which can cause central nervous system disorders such as:

  - Lethargy

  - Chronic Fatigue Syndrome

  - Cold in the extremities

  - Low energy

  - Internal cold

  - Extreme weakness

This means that the life cycle of the worm has begun, and you might need to seek treatment. Of course, this is much more common with longer water fasts, and fasting can actually help you with this condition. However, if you do spot any of these symptoms after completing your fast, it's best to consult your doctor to get the correct diagnosis to move forward and eradicate this. Otherwise, **it might lead to**:

- Intestine obstructions – when a mass of worms blocks your intestines and causes severe pain and vomiting. This is considered a medical emergency and needs prompt treatment.

- Duct obstruction – when a mass of worms blocks the passages to the pancreas and liver.

- Malnutrition – when the worm infestation leads to poor food absorption and causes lack of appetite, slowed growth, and poor nutrition.

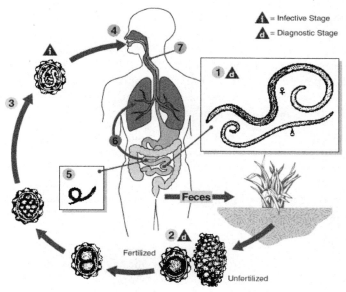

Life cycle of Ascaris Intestinal Roundworm

So as you can see, an enema is actually a very important consideration when it comes to water fasting, and something that you need to think about when you are planning and preparing.

7. Be prepared for the emotional rollercoaster.

Below are **some situations that you might experience while water fasting**, to demonstrate some of the scenarios you might find yourself in. Recognizing these, and knowing what you're going through, will help you if it happens:

Situation #1:

If you get caught up in some uncomfortable emotional turmoil and start asking why, you might think, "That's just the way I have always reacted to these kinds of situations, and it's only worse now because I haven't eaten."

Then a little voice in the back of your mind asks, "Why am I always reacting this way?"

Sometimes, there can be a clear answer, and sometimes there isn't. Either way, relief can often be found in that moment. A long-term pattern has loosened its grip.

It's possible you have asked this question numerous times before: "Why do I react this way?" The difference is now you're fasting. Your mind is clearer and sees through the old fog, it may be unconsciously if it isn't consciously.

Your awareness is heightened, if even for just a moment, to the unreality your mind clings to that is holding you back. It isn't reality; it's only a thought, a recurring idea. Based on something that has already occurred, just like a memory. It might have been something that frightened you. But in this moment, as if by some kind of grace, the dread seems to disappear. This is an opening, a moment of relief. It happens so naturally, unexpectedly, but you can sense something has changed with that brief window of clarity. That "stuck" part of you is now "free."

In a better time or place, this new clarity and comprehension will last for longer than a split second. When these moments begin to happen more intentionally, there can be several similar moments, with the possibility of days or even a lifetime, to practice this new insight and enjoy all its awesome consequences. Exploring this new independence allows us to watch as we integrate this new effort into many areas of our lives.

Situation #2:

Once again, you find yourself in an emotionally disturbing situation and your response is, "It's because I'm so ... [stupid, fat, scared, lonely, undervalued, confused, etc.]." This might be something you've never noticed before; it might be something you've always worried about or thought about yourself. But, because you're fasting, your response might be conflicting.

With your new clarity of mind, you don't have to sit with this terrible feeling, as you might have before. You feel a new kind of lightness, almost like floating over it. This clarity shows you this feeling is temporary, how you're feeling in this moment, that the next minute could be different. You realize that there can be light even when you get surrounded by emotional darkness.

You will "see" how you've created or designed your life with the intent of trying to feel this way. You might come to the realization: "Look what I'm surrounded by; it's no wonder I feel confused." You might even start to reconsider the attitudes, circumstances, and people you've invited not only into your mind, but your life.

And it is in this moment of clarity that you notice how you might have chosen some differently, how a few little things have had a huge effect on you, how making minor alterations and expending a little energy could create space for your true "hidden" potential.

Situation #3:

It's early in the morning, and you open the same kitchen cupboard just like any other day. Today, though, the sight of it is absolutely horrifying. Annoyed, you think to yourself, "Why is this cupboard so cluttered?" The little voice in the back of your mind responds, "Why would I deal with this every single day?" Of course, there isn't an answer.

But then that little voice adds, "Why not tidy this up right now? It should only take a few minutes. And I could feel really good after putting this cupboard in order." Persuaded, because you know that little voice is right, you start straightening that cupboard right then.

Being mindful in the moment, you realize that the act of cleaning is making you feel lighter and lighter, an unnamed heaviness is floating away, that agitated and confused part of your mind is being freed; you're feeling relaxed, even opening up.

Then it becomes clear that you weren't actually aggravated about the cupboard. It is so much larger than that. There was a sense of being out of control, and now you're taking it back. Could it be as simple as throwing stuff out, that clutter of material things? Then you consider the clutter of non-material things. Regaining control can be about disposing of a life stuck in a pattern of constant confusion or agitation. You realize you've chosen something new, embraced a new pattern over the one you were "stuck" in. That can happen so easily when you're fasting.

> "When we fast...the body becomes lighter, more flexible; the mind becomes clearer and more creative. Greater intuitive powers may develop and deep spiritual insights may be experienced..."
>
> Kripalu Center

Exercise and Water Fasting

For a short water fast, it's unadvisable to exercise because you will accelerate your muscle burn, meaning you won't actually burn fat, but will simply feel really bad instead. However, if you're fasting for longer, it's a good idea to introduce some light exercises to help you.

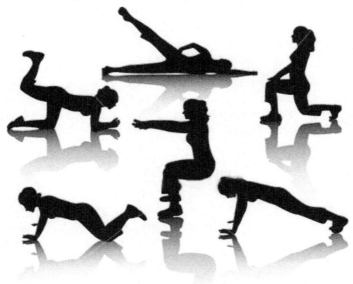

This should be very light cardio-based exercise to ensure that you don't aggravate your hunger symptoms and hurt the healing process. Walking is most strongly advised by health practitioners because it gets you moving but isn't too strenuous. Light jogging and swimming are also ok, but don't go too far because you will end up making yourself unwell.

5 ULTIMATE STEPS FOR BREAKING YOUR FAST THE RIGHT WAY

Breaking your fast in the right way is extremely important to ensure that your digestive system doesn't become overburdened. Here are some tips to help you do this properly:

1. Know what your body has gone through.

During a fast, your body will undergo many biological changes. The work of your digestive system has greatly diminished the production of enzymes, specific to the type of fast being performed. Introducing food back into your diet gradually allows your body the time to re-establish that enzyme production.

Here is a more detailed description of **what areas in your body have been affected**, and **what you need to think about when re-introducing food**:

- The bowels/colon/large intestines: an enema can help you with this, but you will also need to eat carefully and listen to what your body wants.

- The kidneys: drink vegetable and fruit juices, broth, or more water to help the kidneys recover.

- The lungs: introduce light exercise into your daily routine when you feel up to it again to help you feel better.

- The skin: adequate bathing post-fast is critical because one-third of the waste eliminated is excreted through the skin. Use a sponge or a body brush with natural bristles before you bathe.

You will have also been through an emotional rollercoaster with your fast, as water fasting detoxes your mind as well as your body, so you will also need to think about this when breaking your fast. Your brain has been working differently, using other methods to keep your body working, and changing the way it produces hormones. It will need time to readjust back into normal life – although many people have stated that they've changed their thought patterns towards eating after fasting, and only want to each much healthier foods, showing that these psychological changes can become more permanent.

2. Consider how long the transition period is going to be.

The length of your transition period should take twice the number of days of the fast. For example, 10-day fast would require 20 days of commitment and attention.

If you've performed a short fast, your body will readjust more quickly. However, you must be careful not to push yourself too far, too soon. If you've performed a longer fast, you will need to go much slower and think about things on a much deeper level. Never be afraid to go to your doctor for some personalized advice.

3. Think about what you will eat exactly.

You'll need to re-introduce foods in a careful and considered way. Start with easy to digest foods, then move on to the harder, as shown in the list below:

- juices, vegetable and fruit

- raw fruits

- broths, bone or vegetable

- unsweetened yogurt or other cultured milk products

- leafy greens

- vegetables, cooked and in soups

- raw vegetables

- beans and grains

- eggs and nuts

- dairy products

- meats and more solid foods

You will want to avoid anything too harsh on the system – especially in the beginning. This includes salt, sugar, and anything too spicy. It's best to stick to a raw, plant-based diet for at least the first few days. (You will be able to tell how long this should last by the way your body is reacting to new foods. If something doesn't feel right, it probably isn't.) Try looking to the Paleo Diet for some ideas.

Here is **a sample diet plan for you to try for breaking a shorter fast** (between 3 and 10 days). For details on breaking a longer fast, please refer back to the *"30 Day Fast"* chapter.

Day One: Two 8-ounce cups of fruit/vegetable (carrot, some greens, banana, apple) juice that is diluted 50/50 with water 4 hours apart.

Day Two: More diluted vegetable/fruit juice, with bone broth and 1/2 cup of fruit (pears and watermelon) every 2 hours.

Day Three: A cup of yogurt and fruit juice for breakfast, a snack of 1/2 cup of watermelon and vegetable juice, a lunch of vegetable soup and fruit juice, a snack of 1/2 cup of apple, dinner greens with yogurt as dressing, and fruit juice.

Day Four: A soft-boiled egg for breakfast with fruit juice, yogurt and berries as a snack, some cooked beans and vegetables for lunch, an apple and some nuts as a snack, a hardy vegetable soup for dinner with fruit juice.

After this you need to listen to your body to decide what you're ready for. If you've completed a longer fast, you will want to do this slowly and over a longer time period. If you're ready to try bringing in more protein, try moving on to this *sample cleansing diet*:

- Day 1

    - Meal 1: pumpkin pie flavored steel cut oatmeal

    - Meal 2: lettuce wrap including chicken breast, peppers, sliced tomatoes, and mushrooms

    - Meal 3: bean and vegetable soup

    - Snacks: 1 piece of fruit (suggested: apple) or 12 raw nuts of choice (suggested: cashews)

- Day 2

    - Meal 1: vegetable quiche, no crust

    - Meal 2: bean and vegetable soup

    - Meal 3: fresh lentil salad

- Snacks: 1 piece of fruit (suggested: orange) or 12 raw nuts (suggested: almonds)

- Day 3
  - Meal 1: whole grain pancakes with blueberry sauce
  - Meal 2: three-bean and corn salad
  - Meal 3: savory vegetable soup
  - Snack: celery and organic peanut butter

- Day 4
  - Meal 1: egg white & spinach bake
  - Meal 2: savory vegetable soup
  - Meal 3: quinoa and 3-bean salad
  - Snack: apple with natural almond butter

- Day 5
  - Meal 1: fruit and vegetable smoothie
  - Meal 2: quinoa and 3-bean salad
  - Meal 3: balsamic chicken
  - Snacks: raw nuts (suggested: almonds) or banana and 12 walnut halves

- Day 6
  - Meal 1: green smoothie
  - Meal 2: balsamic chicken
  - Meal 3: black bean & vegetable soup
  - Snack: fruit and vegetable smoothie with coconut milk

- Day 7
  - Meal 1: smoothie with cinnamon and apple
  - Meal 2: black bean & vegetable soup
  - Meal 3: skillet chicken breast with quinoa

THE WATER FASTING GUIDE

— Snacks: 1 piece of fruit (suggested: apple) or 12 raw nuts (suggested: almonds)

After you finish your fast – whether it's a long or short one – you will still want to continue drinking at least 8 ounces of water a day. This is a habit that you'll want to keep up always as it helps keep your metabolism working at a quicker speed. On top of this, drinking this amount of water helps your body and mind perform better and fight off viruses and illness!

4. Pay close attention to how your body reacts.

If you experience any adverse reactions to these foods that you're re-introducing to your body, then you need to slow down. Don't do too much too soon, allow your body to dictate you.

If you're breaking your fast too quickly, your body will let you know. You will experience stomach pain, headaches, dizziness, nausea, sickness, constipation or diarrhea – if you experience any of these symptoms, or are worried, then take things more slowly. Everyone must move at their own pace and recover at different times – and you know your body best. If you're really concerned, don't hesitate to go and see your doctor for some advice.

5. Do it slowly.

Begin with smaller, more frequent meals – maybe every 2 hours. Gradually grow towards bigger meals until you are eating normally again. It's also important to chew your foods well because this will aid proper digestion.

78

10 GUARANTEED TRICKS FOR GETTING THROUGH YOUR WATER FAST

Here is **some advice for your water fast**:

1. Commitment

You will need to be committed to your water fast, which is why it's best to pick an ideal time to do it. While doing this, you *will* struggle at times; you just need to get through that. You will learn a lot about yourself and your body as you do.

2. Rest

It's best not to work during your water fast days, as trying to stick to your normal routine will feel impossible and will add unnecessary stress.

3. Keep Busy

Find ways to distract yourself – especially during the hours you'd normally spend cooking or eating. Plan activities in advance, such as:

- Light exercises: walking, yoga, or mild stretching
- Practice breathing exercises to increase lung function and help with detox
- Spending more quality time with your pet
- Make time for prayer or long meditation sessions
- Reconsider old hobbies or passions
- Reconnect with old or long-lost friends

- Start a daily journal to record your fast progress, insights, feelings, and impressions. Keep this journal to use if you water fast again in the future.

4. Get Support

Only tell the people that need to know about your fast — but ensure that they support you on your journey as you will likely need to lean on them. Online forums can also help you find fasting buddies.

5. Again...Be Prepared

I cannot stress enough how important planning is. The more you get ready for your fast, the more successful it will be.

6. Get Ready for Those Weak Moments

Don't fall into your self-doubt. When these negative moments creep up, instead of listening to them, distract yourself instead. Find ways to keep yourself motivated and your spirits up.

7. Don't Stress About Your Colon

Before your fast, it is suggested to eat some high-fiber foods. This will make the first bowel movement after your fast easier. But, keep in mind, that it is normal to not have a bowel movement while you fast.

8. Be Prepared for Dizziness

You may get moments of this, and if you do, immediately sit or lie down wherever you are. This can be due to lowered blood pressure, so give yourself a few moments to recover.

9. Make It Special

Do whatever it takes to make this a special time for you, to help you stick to it. For example, buy yourself a new cup to drink from or give yourself rewards for getting through each day. Anything you might need to keep motivated.

10. Eat Well After Your Fast

When you've finished your fast, introduce foods slowly. Remember that processed foods will not taste good to you anymore, so listen to what your body wants and give it that!

FAQ

1. What can you achieve with water fasting?

Water fasting is a great way to achieve a great number of things; it isn't all about weight loss (although, of course, that is one of the top benefits of the diet!). You can repair and rejuvenate your body, you can help improve your health, and you can end up feeling and looking a *lot* better.

2. How much weight can I lose after a week of water fasting?

The results that you will see will vary from person to person, depending on their bodies, their metabolism, and their lifestyles. People have reported losing approximately 3 pounds a day with water fasting. This goal is within your reach, if you do the fast in the right way.

3. Can you drink tea to detox if you're water fasting?

A true water fast involves consuming zero calories, but this doesn't *all* have to come from water. There are a lot of herbal teas that you can drink to help you detox with a fast – particularly those that use the ingredient *senna*.

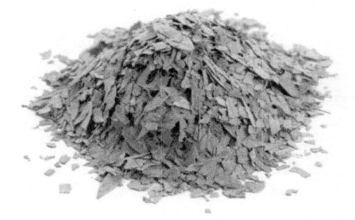

4. Will fasting lead to muscle loss?

Absolutely not. Fasting is actually a really great way to help you build up muscle as long as you keep up your training. You will just need to plan carefully to ensure that you have enough energy to work out when you go to the gym.

5. How does fasting affect your cortisol levels?

Fasting *can* cause a spike in your cortisol levels, which can raise your blood sugar levels. This shouldn't be an issue unless you have an underlying issue in the first place. This is why it's advisable to speak to a health professional before starting a fast.

6. Will your weight return to what it was before if you break fasting?

If you break a fast correctly, and continue to eat healthy and exercise, then you won't have any issues with your weight returning to what it was before. There are some tips on ending a fast correctly earlier in this book.

7. Will your metabolism slow down if you don't eat?

The speed of your metabolism will determine just how much weight you lose overall. Fasting will *not* slow it down. The digestive cleanse that fasting offers actually helps your metabolism to speed up.

8. How long can I do a water fast for?

The ideal length for a water fast is considered to be three days. Any longer than that, and you may wish to consider doing it with the guidance of a healthcare professional. Some people like to do a 24-hour water fast once a week. What you do will depend on your end goal, what you can do, and what you *want* to do. The more a fast can fit around you and your lifestyle, the more likely you'll be to stick to it.

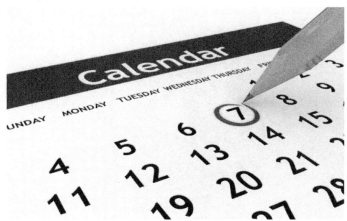

9. Can I exercise when I'm fasting?

Exercising while fasting is actually extremely beneficial. However, doing it on a fasting day where you're consuming no calories can leave you exhausted and very hungry. Fit your workout routine around your fasting for the best results.

10. Should I take supplements when I fast and which ones are best?

A lot of people strongly advise taking supplements when you're fasting to ensure that you're getting all of the nutrients that you need. The most popular ones to use with a fast are discussed earlier in this book – with Branched Chain Amino Acids being the most commonly used and recommended by health professionals.

11. Is it safe for children or older people to do a water fast?

It isn't advisable for children or older people to do a fast. If this is something that you *really* want to try, then speak to a doctor first. They will be able to give you the best, personalized advice to ensure that if you do the fast, you do it safely.

12. Can I fast if I'm slim?

Yes, fasting is not all about losing weight. All you'll need to do is pick a fast that focuses more on the health benefits than the weight loss end goal. A doctor will be able to give you the most suitable advice for you.

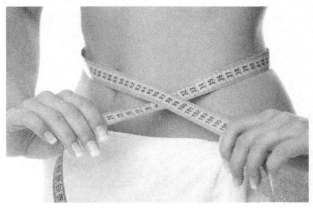

13. Is fasting good for everyone?

There is a small group of people that ***shouldn't fast***. This includes:

- Children
- Elderly people

- Women who are pregnant or breastfeeding
- Those with insufficient kidney function
- People who suffer from diabetes

In fact, if you suffer from any underlying health condition, it's best not to fast without consulting a doctor first. They will be able to tell you what is right for you.

14. How long will results take to show?

A lot of people who have completed a water fast state that they have seen results within the first week. However, it can take 21 days for your body to adjust to your new lifestyle, so it's best to wait for a month to see any changes.

15. Should I only drink water during water fasting?

No. A water fast is all about consuming zero calories for a certain amount of time but that doesn't only have to be with water. You can also include:

- Supplements – to ensure you're getting all the macronutrients that you need.
- Tea or coffee without milk – for a caffeine boost.
- Herbal tea – to help your detoxification.

You will also want to consume healthy, raw foods during your fast to ensure that your system doesn't get all clogged up with the rubbish that was there in the first place!

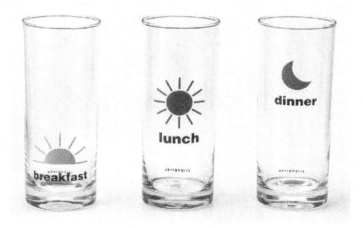

THE WATER FASTING GUIDE

16. Can you water fast if pregnant or breastfeeding?

It's not advisable to water fast when pregnant or breastfeeding as there haven't been enough studies conducted to test how this will affect your baby.

17. Is fasting really necessary?

The answer to this question really depends on you. If you *really* want to lose weight, then this is the most successful way to do so. If you want to lead a healthier, longer life, then fasting is also the best way to do that. If you want to receive the best health benefits from your diet, then fasting is necessary for you.

18. Does the brain not need glucose to function?

No, your brain can also work off of ketones. This is the remaining acid after your body burns its fat for fuel. When your body doesn't get glucose from your blood to power your body's cells, because there isn't enough insulin, it will burn fat instead. This is why fasting helps you lose weight without any effect on your brain!

19. Should I stop my medications when I'm fasting?

If you are taking *any* medications, it's essential that you speak to your doctor before undertaking any fast. That way, you can get the advice that's right for you.

20. Is it safe to fast if you have depression?

Many studies believe that fasting can actually help you recover from depression as it's good for your mental balance. However, it's best to consult a health professional beforehand – especially if you take any medication for this.

21. Won't I become nutrient deficient if I fast?

If you're knowledgeable about nutrients and food, then you will be absolutely fine when you fast. For your metabolism to work effectively, helping you to function normally, you will need:

- Proteins
- Fats
- Carbohydrates
- Nucleic Acids (found in DNA)

Supplements can help you make up anything that you're missing when fasting.

22. How much weight can I lose while fasting?

How much weight you lose when you're fasting will depend on many different factors; your metabolism, the fast that you chose, what you consume on your non-fasting days, and how much exercise you do, to name just a few. Whatever your weight loss goal, you *can* achieve it through fasting.

23. Do electrolytes need to be included in my diet when water fasting?

Electrolytes consist of salts and minerals, such as bicarbonate, sodium, chloride, and potassium, that can be found in your blood. You can get electrolyte-infused water, which can help you with your fast, preventing dehydration and balancing your pH levels to help you feel energized.

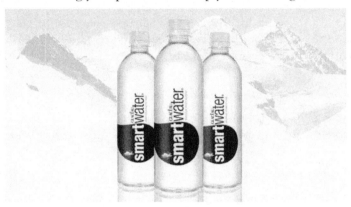

24. How does a water fast trace its roots in religious practices?

Fasting is a practice that be traced back over many centuries and can be seen in almost all religions (Islam, Christianity, and Buddhism, to name just three). This is because it's seen as extremely spiritual because it clears your mind, bringing you closer to God.

25. What should I eat after a 10-day water fast?

Breaking an extended fast, such as a 10-day water fast, needs to be done right for you to stay healthy and maintain the results that you have achieved. After the fast, your stomach will have shrunk, so you will need to be very careful with what you eat. You will want to start with introducing juice, then slowly bring back fruits and vegetables. When you bring food back in, begin with foods that are easy to digest (yogurt, cooked vegetables, etc.) and slowly work your way up to the foods that are the hardest to digest (spicy food and meats). Do this in a way that feels right for you.

CONCLUSION

So now you've gotten all of the information that you need to start your very own water fast. You have all of the tips and tricks you'll need to get started, to stick to the fast, and to end the fast successfully.

By completing this fast, you'll be able to:

- Lose weight

- Get energized

- Become healthier

- Live longer

- Have a stronger mental balance

Those are just a few of the benefits that you'll receive. As you can see from this book, the scientific evidence and the case studies show just how much of a positive impact this diet and lifestyle change can have on your life; so, why not give it a try? You have nothing to lose and a lot to gain.

If you would like to speak to others doing a fast to get the moral support to keep you motivated while fasting, or maybe to ask for some advice, try some of these online forums:

Cure Zone at *www.curezone.org*

The Fast Diet at *thefastdiet.co.uk*

Sometimes, a little confidence boost from someone else who *really* understands what you're going through is all that you need to keep you going.

So, get fasting and good luck!

88

ABOUT THE AUTHOR

Emily Moore has always had a passion for healthy living. It is what led her to study nutrition in university and to constantly be looking for new ways to help people live healthier lives. When she came across the idea of fasting, she was, at first, skeptical. But as she delved deeper and deeper into fasting and learned more and more about how intermittent fasting helps the body and solves many of the most common health problems in today's world, she began to realize the power that this lifestyle has and began working on a protocol to help bring this idea to the average person.

She has thoroughly studied fasting in all its forms, from water, to dry, to intermittent. She practices these types of diets in her own life and has worked with others to help them incorporate it into their lives. As she has done this, she has watched people who have struggled with health issues all their lives become unburdened. She has seen the miracles that fasting can work on the people who do it correctly – that is why she wants to bring fasting to the masses, to help everyone solve their health problems, no matter what they are.